615.534

PG 92

# OPPORTUNITIES IN **CHIROPRACTIC HEALTH CARE CAREERS**

# R.C. Schafer, D. C.
# Louis Sportelli, D. C.

Published in cooperation with the
American Chiropractic Association.

**VGM Career Horizons**

A Division of National Textbook Company
4255 West Touhy Avenue
Lincolnwood, Illinois 60646-1975 U.S.A.

**Photo Credits**
Unless otherwise noted, all
photos appear courtesy
of the various
chiropractic colleges.

# ABOUT THE AUTHORS

At this writing, Dr. R. C. Schafer is president of Associated Chiropractic Academic Press, and has held this position since 1979. From 1973 to 1979 he served as director of Public Affairs for the American Chiropractic Association. He has served as author and/or editor of a large number of texts, manuals, booklets, and articles. Dr. Schafer's texts in this field include:

- *Basic Chiropractic Procedural Manual*
- *Basic Chiropractic Paraprofessional Manual*
- *Chiropractic Health Care*
- *Chiropractic Management of Sports & Recreational Injuries*
- *Chiropractic Physical and Spinal Diagnosis*
- *Clinical Malpractice*
- *Clinical Biomechanics*
- *Developing a Chiropractic Practice*

During the early 1970s, Dr. Schafer served as president of the Behavioral Research Foundation (BRF) of Colorado, a nonprofit educational organization. The firm directed the research and development of training programs, motivational films, and counseling designed to aid career development. In 1971, he served as editor of and authored with others the first training manual for the marketing division of the U.S. Postal Service.

He has taught numerous seminars in the United States and Canada in applied psychology and methodology to both management and lay groups. As author of many papers and programs on personal motivation and achievement strategies, he has made studies in communications tactics and employee behavioral patterns.

Early in his career, he served as director of the Kenmore Chiropractic Clinic in Kenmore, New York, as managing editor of the *New York Chiropractic Journal,* and as a district director for the New York Chiropractic Association.

Dr. Louis Sportelli is currently serving on the Board of Governors of the American Chiropractic Association, and has held that position since 1981.

Dr. Sportelli has authored a patient education booklet entitled "Introduction to Chiropractic" © 1976, now in its eighth printing. Over two million such booklets are in use throughout the world for public information on chiropractic.

He has co-designed and marketed a filtration device for radiation protection. This device, known as the WEDGE Filtration System, has been granted a patent from the U. S. Patent Office. The WEDGE significantly reduces the amount of dangerous radiation to which a patient is exposed during a radiographic examination. This device is used in every chiropractic college in the U. S. and in many private chiropractic facilities.

Dr. Sportelli has also developed and designed anatomical charts for patient education dealing with "whiplash," the lumbar spine, and the cervical spine, as well as producing anatomical charts for the legal profession.

He has lectured extensively throughout the country and

has authored numerous articles for publication dealing with patient management, ethics, radiation protection, public relations, and changes in the health care delivery system.

Dr. Sportelli is a Fellow in the Palmer Academy of Chiropractic Honorus Causa (1984) and has received an honorary Doctor of Humanities degree from Los Angeles College of Chiropractic in 1986. He has received the Meritorious Service Award from the Council on Chiropractic Education in 1981.

Dr. Sportelli has been in continuous practice in Palmerton, Pennsylvania, since 1962. He is married and has two daughters.

# ACKNOWLEDGMENTS

The authors' gratitude is expressed to the following organizations for the reference materials necessary to the development of the manuscript:

- American Chiropractic Association
- Anglo-European College of Chiropractic (England)
- Canadian Memorial Chiropractic College (Toronto)
- Cleveland Chiropractic College (Kansas City)
- Cleveland Chiropractic College (Los Angeles)
- Council on Chiropractic Education
- Federation of Chiropractic Licensing Boards
- Foundation for Chiropractic Education and Research
- Life Chiropractic College—West
- Logan College of Chiropractic
- Los Angeles College of Chiropractic
- National College of Chiropractic
- New York Chiropractic College
- Northwestern College of Chiropractic
- Palmer College of Chiropractic
- Parker College of Chiropractic
- Phillip Institute of Technology, School of Chiropractic (Australia)
- Texas Chiropractic College
- Western States Chiropractic College

# PREFACE

The authors' objective has been to provide an explanation of the field of chiropractic and its opportunities to aid in counseling high school and college students who are considering a health care profession as a career.

As the practice of chiropractic, as well as that of all health care professions, is governed by statutes in each separate jurisdiction, the information offered in this book is general in nature.

The following pages offer basic information on chiropractic as a professional career. Presented in brief form are an overview of the profession, its history and development, the science and philosophy of chiropractic, the basic role of chiropractic physician, career opportunities, educational requirements for the professional degree, licensure information, the professional state of the art, and a look at the projected future of the profession.

The opportunities for doctors of chiropractic are greater today than ever before. Chiropractic offers both men and women an opportunity to serve the health and welfare of our nation and enjoy many material and personal advantages as well.

A career in chiropractic offers the dedicated individual independence, prestige, excellent working conditions, and a rewarding income.

To find a career to which you are adapted by nature, and then to work hard at it, is about as near to a formula for success and happiness as the world provides. One of the fortunate aspects of this formula is that, granted the right career has been found, the hard work takes care of itself. Then hard work is not hard work at all.

—Mark Sullivan

# CONTENTS

of subjects. Incompletes. Class attendance.
Professional attitude and attire. Discipline.
Student guidance and counseling. College
libraries. College laboratories. College clinics.
Student benefits. Student ACA. Student
organizations. College fraternities and sororities.
College honorary society. College athletic club.
Institutional recognitions. Professional
workforce needs. Continuing education.
Considerations involved in establishing a
practice.

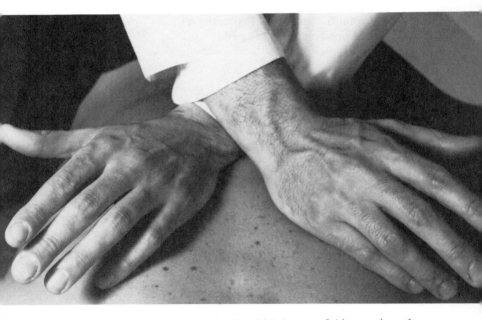

Hands, symbolic of the method by which doctors of chiropractic apply their therapeutic skills to relieve human suffering by the adjustment of the spine. D. D. Palmer, founder of chiropractic, asked one of his early patients, Reverend Samuel Weed, if he knew of a Greek word meaning *done by hand.* Weed offered *cheiro practikos,* and from that word, chiropractic was derived and has remained the name of this drugless healing art throughout the years.

# CHAPTER 1

# AN OVERVIEW OF THE PROFESSION

Chiropractic doctors provide primary health care to an increasing number of patients each year. The doctor of chiropractic serves as a portal of entry into the nation's health care system. The practitioner is concerned with human health and disease processes, considers each patient as an integrated being, and gives special attention to spinal mechanics and the health status of a patient's nervous, muscular, and circulatory systems.

## WHAT IS CHIROPRACTIC HEALTH CARE?

The first step necessary in understanding chiropractic health care is to see how it is similar to the other healing arts and how it is different. First, we should realize that our federal government and all state legislatures recognize three major professions as primary health care providers (doctors who are the first to see a patient suffering a particular complaint). These healing arts, in order of both number of practitioners and public utilization, are the allopathic (traditional medicine), chiropractic, and osteopathic branches of generic medicine.

Governmental recognition, licensure in all states, educational standards maintained by an agency meeting the requirements of, and recognized by, the U.S. Department of Education, inclusion in state and federal health-care programs, and utilization of standardized diagnostic procedures are but a few of the common factors among all recognized healing arts. Although their therapeutic approaches may differ, each healing art is based upon such basic sciences as anatomy, physiology, bacteriology, pathology, biochemistry, and others.

Chiropractic health care is provided for in such federal programs as Medicare, Medicaid, the Government Employees Hospital Association Benefit Plan, the Mailhandlers' Benefit Plan, the Postmasters' Benefit Plan, and included in both the Railroad Retirement Act and the Longshoremen's and Harbor Workers' Compensation Act.

In addition, chiropractic is included in health insurance policies of virtually every major insurance carrier, and in all state Worker's Compensation Acts. A substantial number of major international, national, and local unions (e.g., railroad and rubber workers) and major industrial employers (e.g., General Motors) provide for chiropractic services in their health and welfare plans for all their members and employees.

Second, we should realize that the doctor of chiropractic is primarily concerned with the body's biomechanics—especially that of the spine—and how its interplay with the nervous system affects many important body functions. The chiropractor knows that nerve pressure, or nerve reflex, can cause a disturbance of delicate body functions resulting in an increased susceptibility to disease processes.

The chiropractor is especially skilled in treating nerve, muscle, and skeletal problems such as disc and other back disorders, neck problems such as whiplash, and conditions of the extremity joints. But the doctor of chiropractic can treat much more than these, as attested by the millions of Americans who are chiropractic patients.

Chiropractic is often misunderstood. This is possible because of the profession's conservative approach, which avoids, by its own option, the use of prescription drugs and of major surgery—even though practitioners regularly refer patients for such care when a disorder is considered beyond their scope of practice. Misunderstanding also arises from the chiropractic profession's emphasis on consideration of the whole individual rather than emphasis, as in traditional medicine, on particular symptoms and laboratory findings without consideration of underlying biomechanics.

What is the domain of the science of chiropractic? This is as difficult to define as the domain of chemistry and physics. Any science must be left open-ended or there would be no technological progress. Chiropractic is even more difficult to define because it is such a new science, even though its art of practice can be traced to early civilizations. At this point, we can report the following:

1. There are disorders of the nerves-muscles-skeleton in which chiropractic care has shown outstanding results. This we know to be fact.

2. There are those functional disorders such as certain types of headaches, respiratory disorders, allergies, neuralgias, digestive disturbances, and many other dysfunctions where clinical results are highly encouraging, but further research is needed to define more accurately the scientific principles involved.

3. There are those pathological states for which chiropractic therapy has been rarely involved, yet must remain open to research and clinical study by all the healing arts until adequate solutions are found.

To grasp what chiropractic is and what chiropractic physicians do, it is necessary to offer a simple explanation of the nature of disease, chiropractic's holistic approach, the relationship of structure and function in health and disease, human ecology, and the reasons behind chiropractic's conservative approach.

## STRUCTURE AND FUNCTION IN HEALTH AND DISEASE

The relationship between human structure and function has always been a concern of chiropractic. While it is common knowledge that a diseased organ may cause symptoms to appear in distant parts of the body, chiropractic has demonstrated clinically throughout the years that neurologic insults sited at the spinal column and other areas may cause symptoms to appear in remote organs and tissues. The body is a total being; the nervous system is not a one-way street.

Balance and harmony among body systems result in normal functional tone. This pioneer chiropractic concept is as valid today as it was almost a century ago. Chiropractic contends that this approach must be given the investigation it deserves within all the healing arts and areas of scientific inquiry. It must be placed in practical application, not just offered philosophical lip service, if many of today's health problems are to be solved.

Doctors of chiropractic feel that only when all the healing arts begin to study a patient as a total being in relation to her or his environment, rather than from a purely chemical and organic viewpoint, will health care be able to meet its primary challenges. A comprehensive health care system must be more than an attempt to suppress symptoms by giving drugs or to remove diseased organs by surgery. While a drug may be helpful in easing pain, it does not rectify the cause of the pain. While surgery may be necessary to remove a diseased organ, it does not address itself to the reason that the organ failed to function normally in the first place. The suppression of symptoms or the removal of diseased tissue or organs cannot be considered actions that automatically return a person to optimal health. Chiropractic physicians feel that a comprehensive health care system must be a great deal more than relief, repair, or removal.

## CONSIDERATION OF THE TOTAL PERSON

*Holism* is the theory that the determining factors in nature as a whole are greater than the sum of their parts. A human being is still a mystery even after we add up all the tissues, organs, and systems in the laboratory. Chiropractic recognizes this in its approach to health care.

Our skeletal structure is more than a bony cage to hold our vital organs or a bony hat rack on which nature has hung our muscles. We are more than an assortment of independent organs or a maze of parts. The unifying, coordinating, and controlling forces within the body are essentially the nervous, hormonal, and circulatory systems. There is no organ, tissue, or cell of the body which is not influenced directly or indirectly by these systems. Any dysfunction of one system may have far-reaching effects upon the nervous system because of this inherent relationship.

Structure cannot be separated from function. This is why

chiropractic does not fail to recognize the body's unification. Our bones are more than supports, our muscles are more than pulleys, our nerves more than wiring, and our vessels are more than fluid conduits. Health care must embrace this structure/function viewpoint, in both its gross and microscopic aspects, according to chiropractic principles.

The recognition that the human body has inherent healing powers is common to all ages and cannot be separated from consideration of the body as a total unit. The principle is ancient in origin. What is new to this century is chiropractic's re-emphasis of the doctrines of Hippocrates, the ancient Greek physician. Just as life is defined as the ability to respond to a stimulus, health must be considered the ability to adapt to internal and external stress. To neglect inherent healing forces is to shun natural reserves for recovery.

It would be extremely rare—if not impossible—to find a person ill from a single, specific disease entity such as a stomach ulcer. Obviously, the ulcer is the *result* rather than the cause of the disorder. While surgical removal may be advisable in advanced cases, this does not mean that the conditions allowing the formation of the ulcer in the first place have been removed by the surgery.

It is a rare neighborhood that does not have its share of people who have had numerous operations to remove the numerous by-products of failing organs, while the cause of the failure continues in its nefarious path to be displayed in numerous types of adverse symptoms, signs, and syndromes. Chiropractic believes there must be more to health care than the numbing of pain, the camouflaging of symptoms, or the removal of diseased organs.

Every person is an individual from fingerprints to body structure, function, response, adaptability, habits, and compulsions. All logical theory and therapy should be directed to recognition of individual differences and to the support of an individual's peculiar nature. This is a chiropractic goal.

## WHAT IS THE NATURE OF DISEASE?

All living cells possess irritability, the capacity to respond to external or internal environmental changes by performing special functions to secure proper adaptation and survival. In our body, the nervous system serves as a control system which coordinates cellular activities for adaptation to both normal and stressful external and internal changes and influences. Thus, the nervous system serves a primary role in directing cell function in the never-ending process of adjusting to external and internal conditions.

William Boyd, M.D., in his classic, *A Textbook of Pathology,* reminds us that, "Disease, whether of the heart, kidney, or brain, is disturbed function, not merely disordered structure. For pathology in the modern sense is physiology gone wrong and not just the morphological changes called lesions." In "Disease, A Way of Life," published in *Perspectives in Biology and Medicine,* Stewart Wolf, M.D. states that, "Disease is a reaction to, rather than an effect of, noxious forces."

Thus, disease is the result of normal function out of time and phase with environmental need. It is not the result of any new function. Sickness is not the result of what something does to the body, but what the body does about it because existing mechanical, chemical, and/or psychic irritation of the nervous system prevents adaptation. Disease is not an entity, but a process involving abnormal function and resulting in abnormal tissue changes.

Commonly encountered mechanical irritants include

physical injuries, gravitational and occupational stress, postural defects and faults, developmental imbalances, unbalanced work or play, and deforming changes in the joints. Other irritants commonly encountered in our environment include the toxins of pathogenic microorganisms; drugs, pesticides, and other chemicals; radiation; noise; metabolic wastes; and other pollutants. In addition, the emotional and mental disturbances arising out of the effect of hostile human relations and of the personality's attempts to cope with stress are the principle psychic irritants in our society today.

When a person understands the basic nature of disease, that person will understand why chiropractic places emphasis on the health status of the nervous system. Since one of the basic causes of disease is adverse environmental irritation of the nervous system, it is apparent that any measure that will help to relieve such irritation, regardless of its nature, constitutes indicated treatment. At times, the source of nerve irritation is very obvious, simple, and accessible, making the approach easy. Then again, the irritating factors may be complex, obscure, manifold, and inaccessible, posing a more complicated therapeutic problem.

Obviously, no single therapy offers a panacea. However, one may be better suited to the problem than another, or a combined effort might be advisable. This places an enormous responsibility upon any physician since he or she has to decide which therapy or therapies are indicated for the individual patient.

## HUMAN ECOLOGY

Scientists agree that human beings are infected with a host of viruses, bacteria, fungi, and parasites that are potentially disease producing, but which usually remain latent or harmless. A state of biologic equilibrium between health and illness can be upset by any change in the internal or external environment such as sudden changes in weather, mental stress, overwork, nutritional deficiency, and other factors.

Freedom from infectious disease is not dependent upon the absence of microorganisms, a condition rarely realizable, but rather upon maintaining normal function despite their presence. The body protects itself against harmful microorganisms by producing antibodies and other cell-defense mechanisms to destroy invading microbes and/or their products. It is important to realize that these phagocytes and antibodies are not independent entities. Their role is influenced by the nervous system. Hence, chiropractic contends that the most fundamental therapeutic approach is to assure undisturbed function of the nervous system. Any environmental irritation of the nervous system can upset normal function and permit microorganisms that are already present in the body to initiate an infectious process.

The body's resistance to the invader is not accomplished by one body system, but by all body systems. Such resistance is the accumulated and coordinated forces of the body's totality; some known, some yet unknown.

Health science would be much simpler if a single disease could be attributed to a single cause. But unfortunately this is not the case. We all live in an environment of potential bacterial and viral invasion, but only a minority of us become infected. Even many of the most virulent strains of pathogenic organisms do not infect every person exposed. Bodily resistance, acquired or inherited, and many other factors combine to determine whether or not an invading organism will result in noticeable infection.

Human ecology and economy are complex considerations. The cause of disease is not singular; neither is the response to disease singular. Thus, the logic of a health care program such as chiropractic that considers a person as a total being. Any illness affects the total person, and any disease is multicausal. The total person is affected because illness is not a thing, but a process.

Antibiotics and other potent drugs have certain beneficial effects in reducing bacterial populations. It must not be forgotten, however, that chemotherapy may increase latent infection. As a chemical irritant to the nervous system capable of upsetting the equilibrium in minor infections, the antibiotic could trigger an unfavorable reaction and thus produce complications. Therefore, drugs should not be indiscriminately used in the case of infections of a minor or moderate character. Much is being written today on the subject of iatrogenic disease—a disease that would not have occurred if orthodox chemotherapy had not been prescribed. Old diseases are disappearing, but new ones are appearing which are often man-made—the result of imprudent use of potent therapeutic agents.

*While the chiropractic profession has voiced its concern over the indiscriminate use of the "miracle" drugs for several decades, it has only been in recent years that the scientific community and government agencies have become openly concerned.* The position of the chiropractic profession is not negative, but realistic and positive, compatible with the most advanced facts bearing upon the problems of human disease and disorder. The encouragement of optimum nutrition, fresh air, sunlight, exercise, and personal hygiene long ago became an established routine of chiropractic.

We should be aware that the disappearance of many old diseases cannot be credited exclusively to the healing arts; it is due in large measure to the accomplishments of sanitary engineering. The chiropractor is also a champion of slum clearance and adequate housing and advocates working conditions that avoid unnecessary structural, chemical, and fatigue stress. The chiropractor considers fear campaigns and other well-publicized situations leading to psychological stress a disservice to general health. The practitioner encourages every effort that will decrease poverty or raise the level of living standards, general health, and physical fitness.

Undue irritation of the nervous system is capable of producing abnormal function and thus of initiating disease in the susceptible individual. In broad terms, disease is the result of abnormal function, and abnormal function is the result of the body's inability to cope with stress. Such stress may be the result of any one or a combination of irritations— mechanical, thermal, chemical, hormonal, bacteriological, viral, parasitic, psychological, and so on. Susceptibility is determined by many factors; however, common external factors are environmental changes and virulent organisms, and common internal factors are the body's resistance and hereditary factors.

## HEALTH TRENDS AND STATISTICS

The reason why chiropractic health care is growing in recognition and acceptance, and why it is so important to maintain this freedom of choice of health care, is brought out in public health statistics.

In spite of the rapid advances in science and technology within this century, even the sophistication of traditional medical health care has been unable to meet its most obvious challenges. Illness is far too common, and emphasis is still on after-the-fact care rather than prevention. This was brought out several years ago in an issue of *Newsweek,* where statistics regarding the medical status of the American citizen were revealed:

> The U.S. spends more on medical costs than any other nation in the world. This year alone, the total national health bill will reach $100 billion—about 8 percent of the gross national product of the entire nation. But what are Americans getting for this enormous cost? For all the nation's prowess in the development of sophisticated techniques to detect and treat disease, the U.S. ranks below 20 countries—including Greece, Bulgaria, and Italy—in life expectancy for males. Women in seven countries live longer than their counterparts in America. More important, the U.S. ranks 14th in infant mortality.

Less than a decade ago, the U.S. Public Health Service recognized only 1.5 percent of the nation's 210 million population as being "healthy." Although the United States is the most affluent and technologically advanced nation in the world, these facts underscore the need to analyze many of our traditional and commonly accepted health care practices.

Because of these facts and increasing reports of mounting drug-induced diseases, voluminous reports of unnecessary surgery, rising hospital costs, and malpractice cases, more and more people are turning to chiropractic in search of a more conservative approach. Human ecology, as well as concern for our natural external environment, has begun to receive its due recognition as a major social problem.

While improved sanitation and the development of life-sustaining devices have increased life expectancy in terms of the *quantity* of years during this century, doctors of chiropractic feel more attention must be given to the *quality* of life, from childhood through the senior years.

An interesting comment in this regard was made in the press section of *Reader's Digest* several years ago:

Like the Holy Roman Empire—which was neither Holy nor Roman nor an Empire—the so-called Health Care System in this country is neither Health nor Care nor a System. Today, 95 percent of the medical effort in the United States goes to disease, not to Health; deals with cures, not with Care; and is not a System, but a haphazard conglomeration of medical entrepreneurs—doctors, pharmaceutical manufacturers, hospitals, insurance companies. And the national "health plans" being debated in Congress will, I fear, again be disease-treatment plans, designed to guarantee payment to the treaters. If we do have a Health Care System that is effective in reducing both mortality and disease rates, far less money will be needed than is now being talked about, because emphasis will be on preventive measures and not on still more medicine, doctors, and hospitals.

## CHIROPRACTIC'S CONSERVATIVE APPROACH

Chiropractic, in contrast with allopathic and osteopathic medicine of today, avoids the use of prescription drugs and major surgery. In its approach, it endeavors to establish and maintain optimal body function by correcting abnormal structural relationships and nutritional errors. Chiropractic's goal is to assist the body in such a manner as to enable it to utilize its own biologic reserves for a return to normal function. Its focal point of concern is the integrity of the nervous system.

The doctor of chiropractic has emerged on the scene with a conservative but constructive approach and a rational explanation of the infectious process. At the same time, the doctor of chiropractic recognizes the necessity of cooperating in any and all efforts to save human life by any means available.

As the profession has evolved during this century, it has become increasingly evident that disrelated structures, particularly certain spinal disorders, are a prime source of disturbance to the nervous system and constitute a threat to health not to be ignored.

The chiropractic physician advises and prescribes relative to life-style, habits, and environmental factors that tend to generate adverse influences. Thus, the chiropractor is concerned with the integrity of the entire body. The spinal column and adjacent tissues remain the doctor of chiropractic's primary interest because of their close relationship with the nervous system. However, the doctor's armamentarium may include many more measures other than a corrective structural adjustment of the spinal column and pelvis.

The scientific community realizes today that we have placed too much attention on prescription rather than prevention, too much attention on weakening invaders rather than on strengthening their host. Concern for our internal and external environments should be kept in balance. Ecology concerns both that within and that without.

The healing power of nature is not a new concept. It is a natural phenomenon recognized since the earliest civilizations. The power of the body to resist disease, heal its wounds, and maintain health has always been a fundamental concept in all the healing arts, regardless of doctrine. Unfortunately, this basic concept has been promoted philosophically rather than through widespread practical application. The chiropractic profession has offered important leadership in stimulating renewed recognition that it is the body's true nature to maintain itself in a healthy state and defend itself against most disease forces.

A health disorder is often the result of a disruption of the body's adaptive forces. Such a disruption may be the result of abnormal tonicity. Chiropractic pioneers recognized this almost a century ago. Assisting the patient's natural resistance forces has always been the objective of mainstream chiropractic through corrective structural adjustments, nutritional and physiologic therapies, exercises, rest, and other nontoxic means.

No one healing art offers a simple solution to all the problems confronted in the health sciences. Chiropractic is no exception; however, its emphasis on the importance of biomechanics and body resistance are contributions that have yet to realize their full potential.

## DESCRIPTION OF TYPICAL FUNCTIONS, DUTIES, AND RESPONSIBILITIES

The practice of chiropractic is regulated in all states and in a number of foreign countries. Thus, the scope of practice is necessarily determined locally by existing laws and court rulings in the separate jurisdictions, as it is for all health care professions. The following points offer a general occupational overview for a doctor of chiropractic:

1. During the initial patient interview and consultation, every measure of observation that substantially profiles the patient is employed and recorded.
2. The chiropractor conducts a systematic physical, neurologic, and orthopedic examination using the methods, techniques, and instruments standard in all health professions. The doctor also performs postural and spinal analyses unique to chiropractic diagnostics.
3. Diagnostic roentgenology and standard and special laboratory procedures and tests are used to arrive at a differential diagnosis.

4. The doctor of chiropractic performs or prescribes patient tests, measurements, and evaluations of health status and impairment or disability in establishing or revising treatment programs and preventive programs. The doctor evaluates and updates records to determine case progress and treatment required, and plans the treatment program based upon evaluation of available patient data.
5. The chiropractor corrects, reduces, mobilizes, or immobilizes articular abnormalities, particularly of the spine and pelvis, to normalize structural and functional relationships and relieve attendant nerve, muscle, and circulatory disturbances. These methods do not include the use of prescription drugs or major surgery, thus avoiding the dangers therein.
6. If deemed necessary in case management, the doctor of chiropractic prescribes dietary regimens and nutritional supplements designed to prevent the onset or lessen the existence of some types of dysfunction of the nervous system and other tissues.
7. Physiotherapeutic methods and procedures are frequently used as adjunctive therapy to enhance reception to and the effects of the chiropractic adjustments. Such procedures may include the use of traction, diathermy, galvanic currents, infrared and ultraviolet light, ultrasound, massage, paraffin baths, hot or cold compresses or baths, acutherapy, heel or sole shoe lifts, foot stabilizers, and other modalities common to all the healing arts. The chiropractic evaluates effects of therapy at various intensities and durations during case management and revises therapy to achieve maximum results.
8. First aid, taping and strapping, and other forms of casting are often used in treating injuries of the

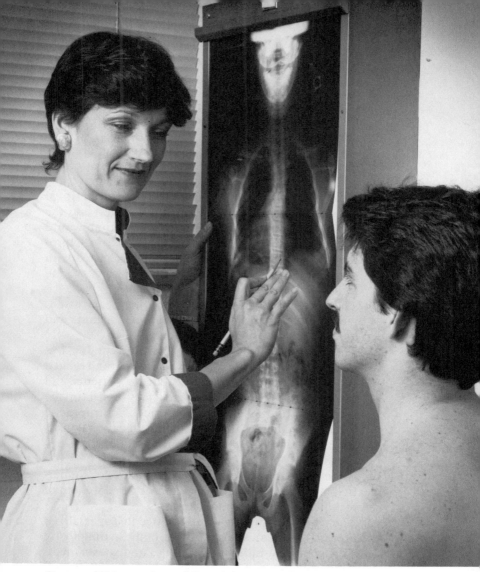

Doctors of Chiropractic carefully explain the structural relationship of the spine to patients prior to beginning treatment. Spinal biomechanics are emphasized; however, age, occupation, weight, and lifestyle are also discussed during the initial patient evaluation.

extremities. Neck, lower back, elbow, knee, and ankle injuries may call for the use of supportive collars, braces, or corsets during recuperation to assist healing and strengthening.

9. Professional counsel is often given in such areas as dietary habits, physical and mental attitudes affecting health, personal sanitation, occupational safety, posture, rest, work, rehabilitative exercises, recreational activities, health habits, adaptive life-styles, and the many other activities of daily living that would enhance the effects of chiropractic health care. Chiropractic care, holistic in approach, is concerned with the total health, welfare, and survival of the individual.

10. The chiropractor orients, instructs, directs, and evaluates work activities of administrative assistants and paraprofessional clinical assistants.

11. The doctor of chiropractic may plan and conduct lectures and training programs on health care and related subjects for chiropractic staff, students, patients, and community groups. The doctor may assist in the teaching, training, and evaluation of chiropractic externs, and he or she may teach in educational institutions or conduct or participate in seminars concerning the basic and/or clinical sciences.

12. The chiropractic physician may plan, develop, or participate in research programs and/or development of technical articles for publication.

13. The chiropractor may limit practice to a specialized area of interest such as orthopedics, diagnostic roentgenology, nutrition, athletics and sports medicine, occupational and industrial health, and attain diplomate status through postgraduate education and certification.

14. The practitioner may be designated *doctor of chiropractic, chiropractic physician,* or *chiropractor,* and may be involved in solo, partnership, group, or corporate practice, or be employed by one or more licensed practitioners.

As previously mentioned, the doctor of chiropractic places emphasis upon the importance of the body's biomechanics, especially that of the spine, and how its interplay with the nervous system affects many important body functions. While specific adjustment of the spine to improve biomechanics and relieve associated nerve disorders is an art developed in contemporary chiropractic, this art has evolved from crude forms of manipulation used quite frequently by ancient civilizations. To appreciate the roots of chiropractic, it is helpful to understand chiropractic's basic heritage.

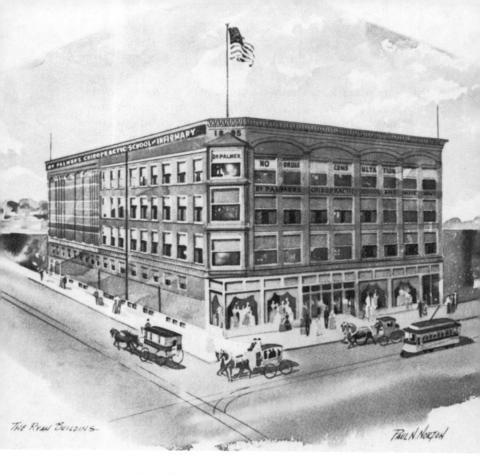

Chiropractic Heritage—where it all began. The photo above illustrates the physical "birthplace" of chiropractic in 1895—the Ryan Building. Dr. D. D. Palmer's office and infirmary occupied most of the fourth floor. Between 1897 and 1902, he began Dr. Palmer's Chiropractic School and Cure.

Chiropractic has its roots in the heartland of America, but the rich heritage of this profession can be found throughout the world as many graduates have returned to their countries to practice this drugless healing profession.

(Reprinted with permission of Palmer College of Chiropractic, Davenport, Iowa)

# CHAPTER 2

# CHIROPRACTIC'S HERITAGE

Generic medicine has its origins largely in magic, priestly practices, and exorcism. Early surgeons bored holes in skulls of the sick so that evil spirits within would be expelled. Sharp-edged stones were the first surgical instruments. Animal masks were used to frighten away demons.

Self-preservation is one of humanity's strongest instincts. Even prehistoric people were concerned with their health, welfare, and survival. Injuries and sickness have always been recognized as a threat to peace and existence, and certain practitioners have been assigned the responsibility of treating disorders of the body and afflictions of the mind throughout the ages.

## IS CHIROPRACTIC A NEW APPROACH TO HEALTH CARE?

Although the exact origin of therapeutic manipulation is lost in antiquity, anthropological findings and interpretation of ancient documents indicate that this health approach has existed throughout the world since the beginning of recorded time.

Some of the earliest indications of manipulation are demonstrated within the ancient Chinese Kong Fou document written about 2700 B.C. Also, Greek papyruses dating back to at least 1500 B.C. gave instructions on the maneuvering of the lower extremities in the treatment of low-back conditions. There appears to be no single origin of the art. Manipulation was practiced by the ancient Japanese, the Indians of Asia, as well as the early Egyptians, Babylonians, Syrians, Hindus, and Tibetans. Manipulative therapy has been practiced by the natives of Tahiti for centuries.

Ancient American Indian hieroglyphics demonstrated "back-walking," in which the ailing would lie down and have their spines manipulated by the feet of others. The early natives of Polynesian Islands had children walk on the backs of the sickly. Observation of therapeutic manipulations by Islanders were reported by explorers in the 1500s.

Some Indian tribes which used manipulative therapy were the Sioux, Winnebago, and Creek Indians of North America. The Aztec, Toltec, Tarascan, Zoltec, and Mayan Indians of Mexico and Central America are also known to have practiced forms of spinal manipulation. The sophisticated Inca Indians of South America are known to have practiced manipulative methods to an advanced degree.

In ancient India, physicians accurately adjusted the spine to relieve sickness, often meeting with marvelous results, and by methods very similar to those used by American chiropractic pioneers in the early 1900s. Egyptian records as far back as 2500 B.C. indicate that they were aware that men and women were stronger when the back was free from unnatural crooks and turns, and accordingly sought to make the spine perfect in form and symmetry.

## EARLY CIVILIZATIONS

Both Eastern and Western cultures had much to do with building the foundation of the healing arts. The Chinese as far back as 2838 B.C. offered great advances with their development of manipulation, massage, anthropometry, acupuncture and acupressure, and moxa, pulse diagnosis, herbs and many drugs. Records are clear that manipulation, massage, and acupuncture were practiced by the Japanese at least as early as 600 B.C.

The different viewpoints among the healing arts today can be traced to their origins in history. Within some primitive societies, it was believed that the one cause of disease could be found in some outside morbid influence that entered the victim. Thus rose the belief in hexes and other evil forces and demons. On the other hand, some societies looked upon illness as an abstraction of the soul from the victim's body. Thus, from these two basic premises evolved the various theories which supported or contradicted the "without" and "within" philosophies which are argued even today among health scientists.

Hippocrates served as chief physician and teacher at the Coan School, located on the island of Cos near Asia Minor. Here emphasis was centered on the patient. Disease was not looked upon as an invading entity such as a demon, but as a vacillating condition of the patient's body—a battle between the illness and the natural self-healing tendency of the body. Although Hippocrates knew the use of many potent drugs, his scheme of treatment was usually confined to assisting nature with mild remedies. Hippocrates founded his teachings on his firm belief that while the causes of disease could be found either outside or inside the victim, "it is our natures that are the physicians of our diseases." He stressed that a human being must be treated as a whole, that the ultimate curative forces are within, that we should study the entire patient and her or his environment, and that we should approach sickness with the eye of the naturalist.

However, all did not accept the Hippocratic approach. On a nearby peninsula, the rival school at Cnidus continued to emphasize the disease rather than the patient. Euryphon, the chief physician and teacher influenced by Egyptian and Mesopotamian cultures, centered his attention on the disease rather than the patient as a whole. He aimed at exact diagnosis and classification and specific therapy, frequently erring by excess detail. He saw the patient's condition only as an "accident" to the patient.

With its prehistoric origins, exemplified in the Coan and Cnidian doctrines, this theoretical conflict has persisted to the present day. The medicine of our own period of ultra-refined diagnosis and highly specialized therapy is largely of Cnidian evolvement. Much of chiropractic's patient-centered and nontoxic approach can be linked to Hippocratic roots.

It should be noted that Hippocrates recognized the importance of spinal manipulation. A prolific writer, he wrote at least seventy books on healing, including *Manipulation and Importance to Good Health* and *On Setting Joints by Leverage*. Emphasizing the importance of the spine, he said, "Get knowledge of the spine, for this is the requisite for many diseases." *Summum bonum*—the highest good—is to remove the cause, taught Hippocrates. Nature must heal; the physician can only remove the obstruction.

In later Greece, Claudius Galen (A.D. 130–200) was the most distinguished practitioner of his time. It was he who first taught the proper positions and relations of the vertebrae and the spinal column and many other features of health and disease. Galen was given the title "Prince of Physicians" after he corrected a paralysis of the right hand of Eudemus, a prominent Roman scholar. He did so by treating the patient's neck, apparently adjusting the neck vertebrae which were interfering with normal nerve transmission to the hand. Galen, like Hippocrates, also recognized the importance of the nervous system when he told his students: "Look to the nervous system as the key to maximum health."

## THE DARK AGES

Humankind's twenty centuries of accumulated knowledge and civilization plunged virtually into oblivion with the fall of the Roman Empire to the barbarian invaders in A.D. 476. This invasion was highlighted by the destruction of hundreds of libraries and their accumulated documentations of scientific achievements. The prevention and treatment of disease took a grave step backwards. Early advances in health care were replaced with omens, superstitions, magic potions, and witchcraft. Concern for sanitation became nonexistent; and ignorance, pestilence, and filth prevailed while logic and science hibernated.

Manipulative therapy also suffered a setback, but the art of spinal manipulation was not completely lost. During the Middle Ages and the Renaissance, the art of manipulation —often called "bonesetting"—was handed down from father to son or mother to daughter and was practiced by at least one person in most communities of Europe, North Africa, and Asia.

Often highly skilled, but without the benefit of formal education, the bonesetters of Europe met with flourishing success. Their success, however, did not meet the general approval of the orthodox medical community. As time went on, the bonesetters of Europe and Asia used manipulative techniques with increasing success, many acquiring great fame as healers. The famous surgeon Sir James Paget wrote, in the *British Medical Journal* of January 5, 1865, an article entitled "Cases That Bonesetters Cure." But even this recognition did little to stimulate objective investigation by the medical aristocracy of the era.

Because of their success with many patients considered hopeless by orthodox physicians, early manipulators were inspired to exaggerate claims of cure which alienated the medical community. Gradually, succeeding manipulators became more clinically and scientifically oriented and less prone to rash claims. But unpalatable memories remained, and members of the medical establishment kept their minds closed to any scientific advances made by the manipulators.

## CONTEMPORARY CONCEPTS

By the late 19th century, most of the basic concepts and clinical principles of modern-day practice had been established. It seems probable that the genesis of the modern theory and practice of manipulative therapy arose from concepts generally acceptable to many 19th-century medical practitioners, since it was during this period that the role of the spinal cord in health and disease was being vigorously explored and discussed. Since that time, however, the three contemporary clinical professions, M.D.'s, D.C.'s, and D.O.'s, have developed in relative isolation from one another. Each group evolved primarily in a clinical setting with a self-generated terminology specific to the history of the particular clinical school of thought.

The conservatism among the traditionists is another reason behind the slow acceptance of any new approach. Any society which does not constantly seek new answers to old problems is destined to become stagnant if not ineffective. It has been the natural history of medical orthodoxy to resist change, often to the point of obstinacy.

Contemporary medical practice emphasizes disease and the results of disease. After proper diagnosis, attention is given to relieve pain and other overt symptoms, repair damaged tissues, and remove destroyed organs. While such an approach has led to brilliant discoveries, much more remains unknown. Neither bloodletting nor transfusion offers the panacea once supposed. On the other hand, chiropractic emphasizes health and the results of normal structure and balanced function. After proper diagnosis, attention is given to seeking out and correcting the causes behind the pain and overt symptoms. Why did function go wrong? What happened to normal tone that allowed pathology to develop? While repair and removal may be necessary and beneficial, it does not remove or repair the cause of the dysfunction by merely removing debris or treating by suppressing the body's attempt to throw off the disease wastes.

Little in life can be logically discussed in terms of black and white. This is especially true within the healing arts. While the chiropractic profession openly recognizes the positive results obtained in the prudent use of chemotherapy, it is also concerned about rigid rituals which fail to consider undesirable side effects. The profession recognizes the need for necessary major surgery, yet is conscious of its dangers. Thus, chiropractic feels that its more conservative approach in a large variety of conditions should be offered objective appraisal before the patient is subjected to potent drugs or the risks involved in surgical intervention. While these measures may be necessary, they should be considered as the last resort and not as the only alternative available in health care.

## THE REDISCOVERY OF CHIROPRACTIC
## PRINCIPLES

During the colonial days of our nation, the majority of doctors were without formal medical education and practiced their healing art along with their other occupations such as barber, minister, or innkeeper. Self-educated lay doctors were typical of the American scene for a long time in those days when few graduates of European universities, who were of the upper social classes, were willing to endure the hardships of the New World. Regular medical education was slow in starting. A medical school was not part of Columbia University until 1860. Apprenticeship or self-training was the usual and almost exclusive path to becoming a doctor in most areas of the country.

Crude forms of preparation for the healing arts existed until long after the Civil War. In fact, it was not until the late 19th century that states began to pass laws licensing the practitioners of medicine.

It is well that we recognize the times as they were when chiropractic was initiated in 1895. The tubercle bacillus (the cause of tuberculosis) was not identified until the 1880s, and Pasteur had established his germ theory as recently as the 1860s. Lister's introduction of antiseptic surgery was still meeting conservative opposition. And it was not until the mid-1890s that X-ray would be introduced in the United States or that Harvey Cushing would bring the first blood pressure instrument to the United States. The mercury vapor lamp and the tuning fork would not be invented until the following year. Yes, medical science was crude; yet there was an air of innovation and many important discoveries and inventions were on the horizon.

It was not until 1919 that matriculants to medical school

were required to have premedical education. As recently as 1930, the only requirement for the licensing examination for the practice of medicine in the state of New York was the completion of four academic years of at least eight months each at medical school.

In the latter part of the 19th century, therefore, the practice of medicine was still in a primitive state; many doctors did not have a regular medical education. American doctors, particularly those in the Midwestern and Western states, were inclined toward nature healing treatments. Some used various forms of diet, herbs and plants, exercise, electricity, purges, bonesetting procedures, religious healing, magnetic healing, sunshine and mineral baths, and other therapies.

Back in 1895, Daniel David Palmer of Davenport, Iowa, was 50 years old. He had been born of English and German ancestry, in the little Canadian town of Port Perry, not far from Toronto. While still young, he moved to the United States. After several occupations—including those of grocer and teacher—he became interested in healing the sick. Because of this interest, he became a student of Paul Caster, an internationally known practitioner of magnetic healing, which was then in vogue. Magnetic healing was a pioneer form of hypnotherapy often used in conjunction with drugless adjuncts and the ancient practice of "laying on of hands."

Palmer practiced his art with unusual success for a period of ten years prior to the discovery of chiropractic. He was an intelligent, yet somewhat eccentric nonconformist, with an intuitive perception of the world about him.

In keeping our discussion in tune with the times, it should be recalled that D. D. Palmer began practice two years before the state of Iowa licensed medical doctors. As a rough-hewn frontier doctor, an intense individualist, his interest in ways to heal the sick led him to be critical of the confusion existing in the healing arts of his day. He felt that many commonly used drugs and potions were actually toxic stresses to patients already weakened by illness. He felt resistance to disease had much to do with the person's functional "tone." In agreement with Hippocratic philosophy, he did not feel that the cause of illness was strictly an agent external to the body, but considered it as a natural response to an abnormal situation. These thoughts were to have a profound effect upon his later life and teachings.

As a self-taught student of anatomy and physiology, Palmer fervently searched for the truth underlying disease processes. In September 1895, he performed a startling experiment. Harvey Lillard, the building's maintenance man, entered Dr. Palmer's office. Lillard was so deaf that he could not hear the noise of the wagons in the street or the ticking of a watch. Palmer inquired about the cause of Lillard's deafness and was told that seventeen years earlier Lillard had suddenly lost his hearing when he strained himself working in a cramped position. Lillard mentioned that at the time of the strain he felt something "give" in his spine immediately before he lost his hearing.

As his usual treatments appeared ineffective, Palmer examined Lillard's spine and found a painful prominent vertebra in the upper spine below the neck which Lillard verified as the spot which hurt when he lost his hearing. Palmer reasoned if the vertebra was reduced, the man's hearing might be helped. Using the spinous process of the vertebra as a lever, Palmer applied a sharp thrust which repositioned the bone. Shortly thereafter, Lillard said that he could hear better than before he lost his hearing! With these encouraging results, Palmer searched for the mechanical laws governing the spine.

With careful study of more patients, Palmer noted that many other types of disorders improved with such "hand" treatments. In search for a name for this new therapy, Palmer asked one of his patients, the Reverend Samuel Weed, if he knew of a Greek word meaning "done by hand." Weed offered *cheiro practikos* and from it the term *chiropractic* was derived. While this term has remained unchanged throughout the years, Palmer was to revise his original definitions of chiropractic many times up to his death, incorporating necessary revisions as the science evolved.

After more clinical observation and investigation, chiropractic became more sophisticated: a formal education program was evolved, entrance requirements by the schools developed, and state laws governing practice were encouraged. However, not unlike many before him who advocated a Hippocratic philosophy, his teachings were controversial among the more orthodox.

## PIONEERS AND EARLY PRACTITIONERS

Palmer's objective was to publicly communicate his concepts about a major cause of disease and his theories about health and its maintenance. His whole-person, "inside" approach was frequently attacked by the members of the medical establishment. Yet the growth of chiropractic theory and the development of its practice depended upon making its basic concepts acceptable to eminent medical practitioners of the times.

Five of the first fifteen graduates of Palmer's teachings were medical doctors, Seeley, Brown, Davis, Simon, and Christonson. William A. Seeley, M.D., was the first graduate of the Palmer institute in Davenport, Iowa. W. L. Brown, M.D., became the first clinic director and journal editor under Palmer. A. P. David, M.D., D.O., became the author of the first three texts to deal directly with the subject of chiropractic. Later, A. B. Hender, M.D., became the first dean of faculty at the Palmer School of Chiropractic. A. F. Walters, M.D., a Philadelphia surgeon and faculty member of the Medical College of the University of Pennsylvania, became a chiropractor who wrote and lectured extensively on his new profession. These learned pioneers perceived that they were initiating a new science of worldwide importance.

Among the early students were Dr. Palmer's son, Bartlett Joshua; Dr. Palmer's lawyer, Willard Carver; as well as members of the older healing arts of medicine and osteopathy. Some of the prominent medical men of the time who became famous chiropractors were J. S. Riley, A. L. Forster, and A. J. Walton. Upon completing their studies with Palmer, these graduates in turn became teachers of chiropractic. Thus, chiropractic was refined as it passed through succeeding classes of students and teachers.

In his quest to communicate this new approach to the nation, D. D. Palmer in 1903 formed a partnership with a surgeon and a homeopath to develop the Portland College of Chiropractic. In 1907, Palmer and Alva Gregory, M.D., formed the Palmer-Gregory School of Chiropractic in Oklahoma City, which at that time was still within Indian Territory.

As early as 1908, Willard Carver had extended Palmer's original concept of joint-oriented nerve interference possibilities to include nerve interference within the osseous grooves in which nerve trunks lie in the extremities, and nerve interference within the vicinity of ligaments, tendons, and muscles. Carver pioneered the use of the then new concepts of mental science and kinesiology. Ever since the early days of chiropractic, the profession has been concerned with nerve interference anywhere in the body, with emphasis on spinal lesions. Chiropractic, however, was never limited only to the spine by either D. D. Palmer or the early pioneers—with the exception of Palmer's son.

D. D. Palmer died in 1913, but not before he had instilled his concepts and enthusiasm for this new science, directly or indirectly, in the minds and hearts of those who would develop the profession into the second largest healing art in the world. For the new few decades, this awakening profession would produce an abundance of martyrs and schools which varied in their expansion, contraction, and interpretation of D. D. Palmer's teachings and writings.

The first state law licensing chiropractors was passed in 1913, the year of Palmer's death, and by 1931, thirty-nine states had given doctors of chiropractic legal recognition. Today, about 25,000 practicing chiropractors are licensed in the fifty states; they are educated in accredited four-year colleges which require a minimum of two years of pre-professional training to qualify for a degree. They must pass basic science and professional examinations as do osteopathic or allopathic physicians.

Spinal analysis and adjustment have always been emphasized within the practice of chiropractic, but they by no means constituted the sole scope of therapy used by the majority of practitioners. In fact, several forms of therapy now gaining popularity within all the healing arts can thank the chiropractic pioneers for their development in this country.

While Chinese acupuncture and acupressure have received much publicity within the popular press since the late 1960s, the use of peripheral stimulation to elicit certain physiologic reactions has been known and commonly applied with chiropractic since its early years.

The use of physiologic therapeutic devices within the healing arts was initiated and developed in this country by the nonallopathic professions, with pioneer chiropractors offering major leadership in both application and development. Physical therapy and the many modalities we know today did not become generally accepted by the medical community at large until the period of World War I, when their use was demanded by the armed services. It is unfortunate that, even today, the application of physiologic-therapeutic adjuncts is de-emphasized in traditional medical education, with practical application generally limited to the rehabilitation ward or to the athlete's locker room.

## DEVELOPMENT OF EDUCATIONAL STANDARDS

Looking back, the importance of quality education was recognized early in the profession. Voluntary efforts to improve chiropractic education were undertaken as early as 1935, when a Committee on Educational Standards was created by the National Chiropractic Association (NCA), now the American Chiropractic Association (ACA).

The Council of State Chiropractic Examining Boards also undertook to improve chiropractic education at about the same time as the NCA, and in 1938 both groups merged into a new Committee on Educational Standards. Under the direction of this Committee, the first college self-study questionnaire was sent to all chiropractic colleges actively engaged in chiropractic education in the United States. As many as thirty-seven institutions of various sizes were in existence at the time. In 1939, the Committee on Educational Standards completed work on educational criteria which were presented to serve as guides for the approval of the chiropractic colleges. In 1941, the Committee on Educational Standards issued its first list of institutions with status, which consisted of twelve provisionally approved colleges. In 1947, the Council on Chiropractic Education

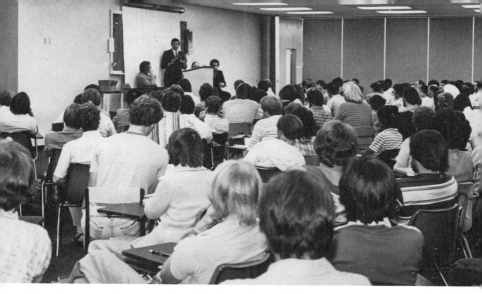

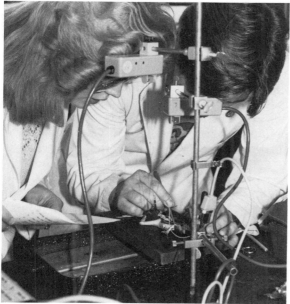

Challenging programs in the classroom and in individual assignments are maintained by the fully accredited colleges of chiropractic.

(CCE) was formed by institutional representatives and members of the Committee on Educational Standards.

During the twenty-year period from 1941 to 1961, the Committee continued to function to strengthen chiropractic education. Many of the weaker institutions were merged with other institutions to create stronger academic programs. A number of the grossly substandard institutions were simply closed. By 1961, the number of colleges had been reduced to ten. In 1964, the NCA merged with other groups to form the American Chiropractic Association which continues to support the goals of the CCE. In 1971, the CCE was incorporated as an autonomous national organization and continues to function as such today.

Recognition by the U.S. Office of Education did not come easily. Initial contact with the USOE by the CCE was made in 1952, with an official application for recognition being filed in 1959. Suggestions for strengthening academic status and procedures were received and implemented, and in 1969, an unofficial filing of materials was made with the USOE which resulted in further suggestions for change. In August 1972, the CCE filed its formal application with the USOE, which resulted in the initial listing of the CCE as a "nationally recognized accrediting agency" by the U.S. Commissioner of Education, Department of Education. Periodically, recognition of the CCE has been renewed by the Commissioner.

## THE NATIONAL BOARD OF CHIROPRACTIC EXAMINERS

Since its formation in June 1962, the National Board of Chiropractic Examiners (NBCE) has shown a steady growth in acceptance and stature. The first three years of the Board's existence were spent in establishing proper guidelines for the organization, defining the purpose and areas of activity for the National Board and consulting with several of the state chiropractic examining and licensing boards to determine how the Board could best serve and assist these licensing bodies. Much attention was given to the organization and purposes of national boards in the other healing arts in order to profit from their experience.

During the formation of the Board, the Council of State Chiropractic Examining Boards, an organization made up of chiropractors and officials serving on state licensing boards, the presidents and faculty members of chiropractic colleges throughout the nation, and the General Committee of the Profession on Education cooperated to formulate the basic organization of the NBCE.

The first National Chiropractic Board Examination was held in 1965. By 1967, the examination was being administered to 825 individuals in seven testing centers across the nation. By the mid-1970s, both the number of individuals being examined and the number of examination sites had multiplied substantially.

The vast majority of Chiropractic Licensing Boards and about half the Basic Science Examining Boards recognize diplomates of the examination offered by the National Board of Chiropractic Examiners. Because of the student benefits involved in meeting a broad criteria for licensure, many chiropractic colleges presently consider passing the National Board's examination a requirement for graduation.

The executive headquarters of the NBCE is located at 1610 29th Avenue Place, Greeley, Colorado 80631.

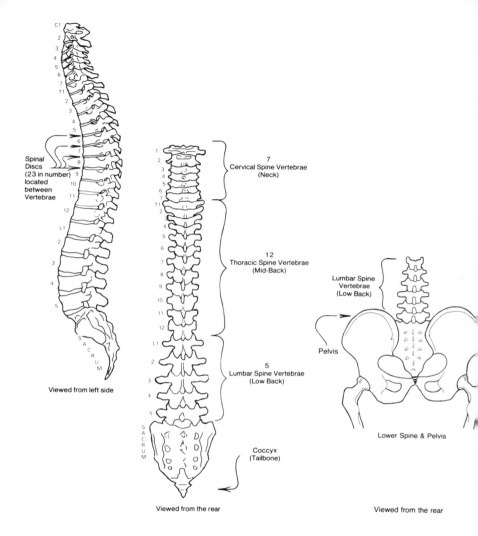

**Spinal Discs** (23 in number) located between Vertebrae

Viewed from left side

7 Cervical Spine Vertebrae (Neck)

12 Thoracic Spine Vertebrae (Mid-Back)

5 Lumbar Spine Vertebrae (Low Back)

Coccyx (Tailbone)

Viewed from the rear

Lumbar Spine Vertebrae (Low Back)

Pelvis

Lower Spine & Pelvis

Viewed from the rear

### What Does a Doctor of Chiropractic (D.C.) Do?

All doctors use a standard procedure of examination to diagnose a patient's condition in order to arrive at a plan of treatment. The examination of the spine to evaluate structure and function is what makes chiropractic different from other health care procedures. Minor displacements or derangements causing irritation directly to spinal nerves or by pressure indirectly through reflexes may cause malfunctions in your body.

# CHAPTER 3

# BASIC ROLE OF THE CHIROPRACTIC PHYSICIAN

The practice of chiropractic is recognized and regulated by all fifty states and Puerto Rico as an independent health service. The profession has proven its value as a public health service. As long ago as 1929, the Congress of the United States passed a law for licensing doctors of chiropractic in the District of Columbia.

On foreign shores, the practice of chiropractic is officially recognized and regulated in provinces of Canada and in Switzerland, West Germany, New Zealand, Western Australia and Bolivia, and is acknowledged and accepted in the British Isles, South Africa, Zimbabwe, Japan, France, Denmark, Belgium, Italy, and some parts of the Middle East.

## THE SCIENCE OF CHIROPRACTIC

Traditionally, science has been regarded as classified or systematized knowledge. The intent of science is the acquisition of truth. It deals with facts and propositions verifiable by objective evidence.

In a broader sense, however, science is more than classified knowledge. It is an attitude of objective inquiry, a method of investigation, and a process of reasoning which guides the inquiry and controls the interpretation. It organizes isolated facts into meaningful relation with each other and arrives at a synthesis within the largest possible frame of reference. This indeed is the supreme goal of science. Nothing better illustrates this process than the various factors out of which developed the branch of science known as chiropractic.

First, chiropractic is a body of classified knowledge. The essentials of the basic sciences form the nucleus of chiropractic education. From these come the data which support the theory of chiropractic and shape the practice. Such knowledge is supplemented by additional knowledge garnered from chiropractic centers in various parts of the world.

Second, chiropractic represents the typical attitude characteristic of science. There is within chiropractic an insatiable curiosity concerning the phenomena with which its practitioners deal. There is a willingness to modify any theory when more tenable explanations are advanced and to abandon error when error is shown to exist. In any science, the ideas and theories of predecessors must be preserved only insofar as they represent the present state of science. There is also a definite disposition to demonstrate the efficacy of chiropractic by subjecting it to comparative evaluation, using other therapies as controls.

Third, the methods of obtaining data in chiropractic are the methods of science. These include observation, description, experimentation, statistics, and prediction.

*Observation and Description.* No other health care profession has made such elaborate, detailed, and exact description of the facts of anatomical disrelation. In daily practice, the doctor of chiropractic is occupied with the details of body mechanics and carefully records the findings. The doctor of chiropractic has developed precision methods in radiography to render findings objective, measurable, and intelligible to the scrutiny of others. He or she has utilized photography and mechanical devices for the study of posture, and has employed standard techniques of diagnosis in gathering data on which to base conclusions relative to the applicability of chiropractic to specific conditions. Technical equipment has also been designed and produced for the study of the statics and dynamics of the body, particularly of the vertebral column and sacroiliac mechanisms.

*Experimentation.* It will be recalled that chiropractic began with an experiment. Now chiropractic research uses experimental methods to determine and explain the relation of particular kinds and degrees of anatomical disrelation to specific pathological processes and symptoms and has acquired an immense body of data in this way. Experiments have varied the technique of corrective adjusting to discover the unique measures most efficient or best adapted to certain conditions and types of patients. Special experiments have checked the immediate effect of the adjustment upon heart rate, blood count, blood pressure, and other physiological phenomena. Other experiments have measured the extent to which a correction at one spinal level alters the status at another level.

*Statistics.* A far-reaching program of statistical research is in progress within accredited chiropractic colleges and agencies of the American Chiropractic Association to evaluate the results of chiropractic therapy in specific types of cases.

Chiropractic is stringently bound by the rules of logic. It reasons by induction and deduction, applies the methods of establishing causal relationships, and follows accepted procedures in formulating hypotheses and theories.

In this text of 1910, Dr. Palmer states that, "Chiropractic is a science, not a building; it was created, not built. Its foundation is not that of principles. It is founded on anatomy— osteology, neurology, and functions. It is not built out of principles as a mason would build a house out of brick. Chiropractic is a science—a knowledge of health and disease reduced to law and embodied into a system . . . "

It was only natural, as is the case in all new professional efforts, that the pioneers of chiropractic had to seek their way by trial and error. Lacking the guideposts of precedent and an adequate body of scientific data, they had to forge new procedures and grope for satisfying interpretations of the as-yet-unexplained phenomenon of their clinical success. Consequently, there was the tendency during the early years both to oversimplify the rationale and to miss the full biological implications of the measures employed.

These trends have their parallels in the history of the other schools of healing, especially during their formative, strictly empirical phases. One may recall the futile efforts of traditional medical practice to discover a bacterial cause for almost all disease during the early days of bacteriology.

Today's chiropractic profession recognizes that it shall be governed by the requirements of science. It is fully aware that in all human attempts to restore and maintain health there are intangible factors which defy scientific investigation and explanation, but until these obstacles have been overcome we must leave these matters to logical hypotheses. However, chiropractic is a part of science in that it utilizes in the most meticulous way the scientific achievements provided by all relevant sciences to explain the phenomena of health and disease. It also uses a scientific methodology to pursue further investigation in this field.

## BASIC PRINCIPLES OF PRACTICE

Chiropractic, regardless of jurisdiction, is built upon three related scientific theories and clinically established principles. Although these theories have been refined over the years, they represent in essence the basic concepts established by chiropractic pioneers early in this century. Today, they are accepted premises within the scientific community.

*Disease may be caused by disturbances of the nervous system.* While many factors impair human health, disturbances of the nervous system are among the most important factors of disease etiology. The nervous system coordinates cellular activities for adaptation to external or internal environmental change. Environmental agents and conditions which unduly irritate or inhibit the nervous system, and to which the body cannot successfully adapt, produce fluctuations in the pattern of nerve impulses which deviate from the norm. Thus originate many diseases.

*Disturbances of the nervous system may be caused by derangements of the musculoskeletal structure.* Spinal and pelvic derangements (subluxations) or the loss of spinal mobility is a common clinical finding in the human body. These derangements may cause irritability within the nervous system and interfere with normal nerve supply. Oftentimes this is caused by stresses and strains arising within the musculoskeletal system due to the human attempt to maintain this erect posture. The mechanical lesion, or subluxation, is a common result of gravitational strains, asymmetrical activities and efforts, and developmental defects or other mechanical, chemical, or psychic irritations of the nervous system. Once produced, the lesion becomes a focus of sustained pathological irritations which may trigger a full-fledged syndrome of severe nerve-root irritation.

*Disturbances of the nervous system may cause or aggravate disease in various parts or functions of the body.* Vertebral and pelvic subluxations may be involved in common functional disorders of a visceral and vasomotor nature and, at times, may produce phenomena that relate to the special organs. Under predisposing circumstances, almost any component of the nervous system may directly or indirectly cause reactions within any other component by means of reflex mediation.

A human being is a total integrated entity. A disorder in a specific organ or tissue will have its effect upon other functions, organs, and tissues. In addition, we should be mindful that a combination of independent causes of bodily dysfunction may jointly have more serious debilitating effects than one cause might have had separately. For example, vertebral subluxation or fixation may be one of the contributions to the triggering of migraine headaches, asthmatic syndromes, and certain types of neurovascular and neurovisceral instabilities. Often, correction of the spinal lesion is a very important step toward effective total management of the case.

## DIAGNOSTIC AND THERAPEUTIC METHODS

In general, diagnosis plays the same role in chiropractic as in all the healing arts; it is the basis for determination of the treatment. A chiropractic diagnosis is arrived at after an interview, physical examination, and the use of diagnostic aids and laboratory tests.

The initial interview and consultation with the patient is of utmost importance. Every measure of observation that will more substantially profile the patient is employed and recorded. The doctor of chiropractic conducts a systematic and thorough physical examination using the methods, techniques, and instruments that are standard with all health professions. In addition, he or she includes a postural and spinal analysis, an innovation in the field of physical diagnosis and examination.

The chiropractic physician, using the standard procedures and instruments of physical and clinical diagnosis, is well acquainted with the need for differential diagnosis. Diagnostic radiology, especially as it relates to the skeletal system, is a primary clinical diagnostic aid in chiropractic—and has been since the early 1900s.

In addition, doctors of chiropractic are knowledgeable in the standard and special clinical laboratory procedures and tests usual to modern diagnostic science. Each accredited college has a laboratory licensed to carry on clinical laboratory examinations in such fields as cytology, chemistry, hematology, serology, bacteriology, parasitology, and electrocardiography.

Chiropractic treatment methods are determined by the scope of practice authorized by state law. In all areas, however, these methods do not include the use of prescription drugs or major surgery. Essentially, treatment methods include chiropractic adjustment, dietary advice and nutritional supplementation, physiotherapeutic measures, and professional counseling.

The most characteristic aspect of chiropractic practice is the correction (reduction) of a subluxated, hypermobile, or fixated vertebral or pelvic segment(s) by means of making a specific, predetermined adjustment. The purpose of this correction and its determination is to normalize the relationships of segments within their articular surfaces and relieve the associated nerve, muscle, and circulatory disturbances.

Vitamin and mineral food supplements can, if professionally supervised, serve to prevent the onset of some types of dysfunction of the nervous system and other tissues. If deemed necessary in case management, dietary regimens and nutritional supplements are often advised as adjunctive therapy.

Physiotherapeutic methods and procedures are frequently used as adjunctive therapy to enhance the effects of the chiropractic adjustments. Such procedures may include the use of diathermy, galvanic currents, infrared and ultraviolet light, ultrasound, traction, paraffin baths, hot or cold compresses, acutherapy, hydrotherapy, heel or sole lifts, foot stabilizers, and other commonly utilized modalities. Taping and strapping and other forms of treatment are often used in injuries of the extremities. Neck, lower back, elbow, knee, and ankle injuries may call for the use of supportive collars and braces to enhance the effects of corrective treatments and to assist healing and strengthening. Rehabilitative exercises, as a physical therapy, comprise an important aspect of professional counseling to assist recovery and prevent further strain.

Counseling is often given in such areas as nutrition, physical and mental attitudes affecting health, personal sanitation, occupational safety, lifestyle, posture, rest, work, and the many other activities of daily living which would enhance the effects of the chiropractic adjustment. Chiropractic is truly concerned with the total individual: the patient's health, welfare, and survival.

Professional councils on roentgenology, orthopedics, nutrition, and diagnosis and internal disorders strive to keep the field abreast of the latest scientific and technological advancements. Councils on mental health, neurology, technic, physiological therapeutics and sports injuries are continually investigating even more efficient methods of treatment.

## PHILOSOPHY OF CHIROPRACTIC

The science of mechanical forces as they are applied to a living organism is called *biomechanics*. This study includes those forces that arise internally such as during a strain or locomotion or externally such as from a blow to the body or by gravity. The term *biodynamics* refers to the scientific study of the nature and determinants of an organism's behavior during motion.

The relationship of biomechanics to biodynamics has been emphasized by the chiropractic profession for almost a century, yet there is still need for more objective research to support clinical observations. Evidence of the importance of removing and preventing spinal subluxations and fixations is growing each year, as the nervous system maintains a primary role in integration of all body systems.

The central nervous system originates in the brain centers and extends down through the spinal column, reaching every part of the body through the peripheral nervous system. Interference anywhere in the nervous system impairs bodily functions and induces disease. One site of insult is that point where nerves exit or enter the spinal column. Such insults result in what chiropractors term subluxations (partially displaced vertebrae) or fixations (partially restricted vertebrae) which in turn cause or contribute to neurological disorders affecting both structural balance and functional tone.

The mechanical lesion, a subluxation or fixation, is an attending complication of those mechanical, chemical, and/or psychic environmental irritations of the nervous system, which in the human body produce muscle contraction sufficient to cause dysfunction of the spinal articulations. Once produced, the lesion becomes a focus of sustained irritation. It irritates nerves in the articular capsules, ligaments, tendons, and muscles of the involved spinal segment. A barrage of impulses streams into the spinal cord, where they are received and relayed to motor pathways for conduction to muscles and glands, initially in excessive amounts. The contraction which originated the lesion is thereby re-enforced, perpetuating both the subluxation and the pathological process which it engenders. This phenomenon is commonly termed the vertebral subluxation complex.

Not all the irritation originates this way, however. The microtrauma attending the vertebral subluxation may set off an inflammatory reaction with swelling which tends to encroach upon a portion of the spinal nerve. The process may even terminate in adhesions.

Each of the vertebrae of the spine are separated from each other by a spinal disc. These twenty-three pad-like structures not only cushion the twenty-four movable spinal vertebrae, but also make possible the flexibility of the spine which is essential to normal movement. Under certain conditions, disc disorders may lead to involvement of the spinal nerves directly or indirectly. With the contributory factor of the subluxation, such complications may trigger a full-fledged syndrome of severe root compression or irritation.

While such mechanical lesions are most often associated with the spine, studies have indicated that they frequently exist in other parts of the musculoskeletal system. The musculoskeletal system is intimately connected with all other systems through the nervous system.

## THE ART OF CHIROPRACTIC

Corrective structural adjustment by a chiropractic physician should not be confused with other forms of manipulation. Manipulative therapy in one form or another is used in

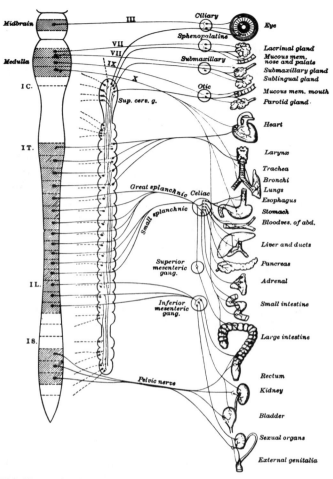

This illustration is taken from Gray's Anatomy, a standard textbook recognized and widely used in the leading schools of medicine, osteopathy, and chiropractic. It shows the nerve supply to the vital organs from the brain and spinal cord and suggests the need for maintaining uninterrupted communication through the nerves.

The illustration helps to show that every vital organ in the body is connected with and controlled by nerves from the spinal cord and brain. Through this knowledge, one can more fully understand why chiropractic treatments can relieve so many human ailments.

[Reprinted with permission from Clemente, Carmine D. (editor): Gray's Anatomy. Lea & Febiger, Philadelphia, 1985.]

varying degrees in all the healing arts. Allopathic manipulation is usually little more than putting a joint through its normal range of motion, by a therapist, in order to stretch muscles and break adhesions. Osteopathic manipulation is designed to increase joint motion and relieve fixations. On the other hand, a chiropractic corrective adjustment is made only after careful analysis, delivered in a specific manner, to achieve a predetermined goal. It is a precise, delicate maneuver, requiring special bioengineering skills and utilizing a "short lever, high velocity" thrust. The process is seldom painful.

Most chiropractic corrective adjustments are made upon the joints, especially those of the spinal column. Some techniques, however, are light-touch reflex adjustments which involve the nerves of the body's blood vessels, lymph vessels, and muscles. These surface techniques are far more than massage or trigger-point releases, for they must involve careful diagnosis and be scientifically applied after comprehensive chiropractic training.

## CHIROPRACTIC PATIENTS

There were about 4,250,000 chiropractic patients in the United States in 1964, or about 2.2% of the entire population. By 1974, the number had increased to over 7,500,000 patients, or 3.6% of the population. This 77% increase in the number of patients occurred while the general population grew only by 10.4%. New chiropractic patients totaled at least 9,500,000 in calendar 1982. During the period from 1969 to 1981, the proportion of the United States population that had seen a chiropractor at least once rose from 20% to

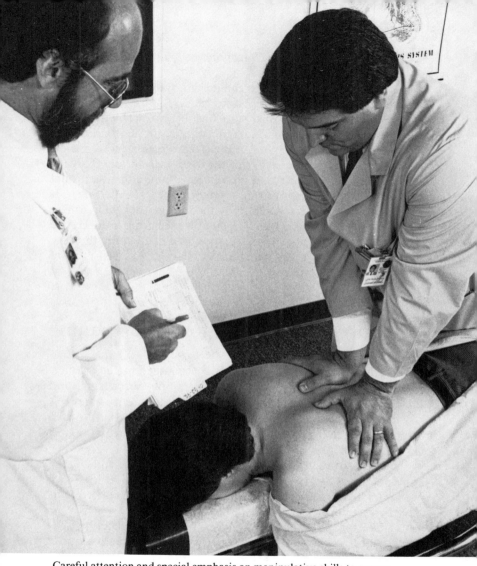

Careful attention and special emphasis on manipulative skills to ensure the highest degree of expertise necessary to perform the various procedures utilized in spinal manipulation. Manipulation is a personal art form, and doctors of chiropractic have excelled in developing specific technics to improve the effectiveness of chiropractic spinal adjusting.

almost 40%. According to the growth pattern, such figures would be substantially higher today.

According to the latest statistics, health problems classified as neuromusculoskeletal account for 82% of all conditions treated. Other conditions treated, in order of their frequency, are those involving the function of internal organs (12%), blood vessels and circulation (5%), and nutritional deficiencies or disorders of nutrient utilization (0.7%).

Several surveys taken both within and without the profession have indicated that there is no measurable difference between chiropractic patients and those of any other healing art relative to age, sex, occupation, income status, education, or any other social factor.

## PROFILE OF A TYPICAL DOCTOR OF CHIROPRACTIC

The typical practicing doctor is a married male. The percentage of female practitioners is rapidly increasing, and today approximately 25% of the student enrollment is female. The typical doctor is 37 years old and has a 50% chance of living in a city with a population of over 50,000. He or she has been in practice about 10 years.

In addition to graduation from a chiropractic college, the doctor has attended a college or university for at least two years, majoring in premedicine or the physical and biological sciences.

The typical doctor was 27 years old when receiving the doctorate degree. He or she is qualified to practice under state law in all states through examination before state boards. The doctor is actively involved in postgraduate education, either at the colleges themselves or through state and regional seminars.

The majority of doctors of chiropractic are in solo practice, although those involved in some form of group practice now comprise more than one-quarter of the total. The typical doctor's office is located in a neighborhood business district, has been there for eight years, and employs two assistants.

The typical doctor of chiropractic practices 4.2 days each week, in which he or she attends to the needs of 116 patient visits. The chiropractor's income and lifestyle are typical of those enjoyed by other primary health care providers.

The typical doctor is a member of national, state, and district professional associations. He or she is also an active and contributing member of local community and civic groups. The doctor has a position of responsibility to patients and community and uses professional abilities conscientiously and with integrity to serve those who depend upon her or him for proper health care and advice.

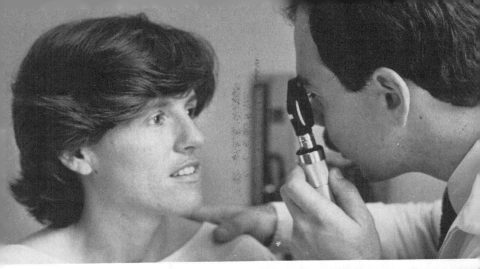

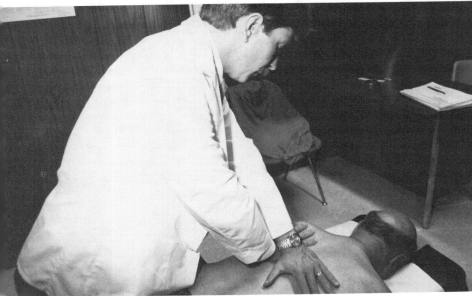

A comprehensive consultation, thorough physical examination, and complete postural and structural evaluation is performed by the doctor of chiropractic prior to beginning treatment. Specially designed equipment for specific spinal adjustments are used to insure maximum therapeutic benefit as well as patient comfort.

# CHAPTER 4

# CHIROPRACTIC AS A PROFESSIONAL CAREER

Increasingly wide acceptance and a rapidly growing population make the future of chiropractic a boundless one. Chiropractic is a rapidly growing profession offering a career of rare opportunity and service to the dedicated doctor. In return, the profession provides security, prestige, and excellent income to its practitioners.

## WHAT ARE THE CAREER OPPORTUNITIES?

According to census figures and a survey made by the American Chiropractic Association, there is approximately one doctor of chiropractic serving every group of 10,000 people in the United States. A more desirable ratio would be one doctor of chiropractic for every 4,000 people. Thus there is an urgent demand for an immediate increase in the number of doctors of chiropractic in the United States, Canada, and several foreign countries. Literally hundreds of towns that could adequately support a doctor of chiropractic are without one. Few cities of any size—even the largest—have enough doctors of chiropractic in ratio to the population.

Not only is chiropractic among the least crowded of all professions, each year expanded service opportunities are opened to those in the profession. For instance, more companies are referring accident cases to the doctor of chiropractic for fast and efficient treatment of injuries involving the back, extremities, whiplash, and other joint damage. Experience has shown that both personal and economic benefits accrue when chiropractic treatment returns a patient to active life more quickly.

To expand its area of service and assure continued opportunities for the profession, chiropractic is engaged in several research programs. Research is being done in relation to low-back pain, headaches, arthritis, rheumatism, nervous disorders, and many other health afflictions. In addition, special X-ray research is being carried out to develop safe procedures to decrease industrial injuries and structural abnormalities. Research and development have identified new areas of need for the doctor of chiropractic and will no doubt provide many more new opportunities in the future.

## GENERAL PRACTICE

Chiropractic is a broad field. The clinical practice of chiropractic has proven applicable in a wide variety of diseases and disorders. The doctor of chiropractic is a particular kind of physician. As such, he or she is engaged in the treatment and prevention of disease and in the promotion of public health and welfare. With the advances made by chiropractic science in the field of biomechanics, a doctor of chiropractic will find wide areas of service open as a general practitioner or as a specialist within the field.

The vast majority of chiropractic physicians feel that general practice offers the greatest inducements and rewards. In general practice, a doctor of chiropractic is given the opportunity to use the full scope of his or her professional preparation.

Because of the increasing complexities in health care and the rapid technological advances in chemotherapy and surgical procedures, more and more allopathic and osteopathic practitioners are entering the specialties, leaving a dire need for the general practitioner, especially in rural communities. Increasingly, we find that chiropractic physicians are fulfilling the role of family doctor. The reason for this is threefold: first, the chiropractor's approach to the patient as a total being; second, the fact that more than 50 percent of chiropractic doctors are located in rural and suburban areas; and third, because the doctor/patient relationship under chiropractic care is often more personal. A recent study substantiated this latter point.

In 1974, the Department of Family and Community Medicine of the University of Utah College of Medicine conducted a comparison of the effectiveness of the allopathic physician and chiropractic care. The study showed, both in terms of the patients' perception of improvement in functional status and of patient satisfaction, that the chiropractors appear to have been as effective, if not more effective, with the patients they treated as were the allopathic physicians. The two groups of patients under investigation and comparison were not significantly different with regard to age, sex, race, education, marital status, income, hypochrondria, or attitudes about the medical profession in general.

The majority of newly graduated chiropractors prepare for

private practice by associating themselves with well-established general practitioners on a salary or income-sharing basis. Others become staff members in group practices where there is a growing demand for qualified professional personnel. Due to the rising costs of office equipment, furnishings, and facilities, association with an established practice offers an opportunity to enter practice without a large financial investment.

## SPECIALTIES

While it is true that the majority of doctors of chiropractic choose general practice, there is ample opportunity within the profession for development in a special field of interest. A chiropractic physician may choose to specialize in orthopedics, roentgenology, sports medicine, pediatrics, independent disability evaluations and nutritional consultation, or other special areas of interest. Many doctors of chiropractic have had outstanding success in their selected fields of specialty. This is particularly noteworthy since there has been a trend in recent years towards specialization in all the health professions, especially in practices located in highly populated urban areas.

An increasing percentage of chiropractic physicians devote their entire practice to chiropractic roentgenology (the taking and interpreting of diagnostic X-ray films for the general practitioner) or chiropractic orthopedics (the specialty concerned with the preservation and restoration of the function of the skeletal system, its articulations, and associated structures). The ACA councils on roentgenology, orthopedics, sports injuries, and nutrition have designated programs leading to certification and diplomate status within the specialty, requiring several years of postgraduate training.


## TEACHING AND RESEARCH

For those whose interests and talents qualify them, there is excellent opportunity to teach in chiropractic colleges in the United States, Canada, England, and Australia. This is a most rewarding way of expressing chiropractic skills. With the demand for doctors of chiropractic increasing so rapidly, qualified teachers serve an increasingly important role in broadening the profession.

Research has also become a vital part of chiropractic advancement, just as it must in all modern health care professions. Research is vital to the profession today, and many dedicated individuals are considering this career to contribute to the advancement of the profession and the general public welfare. The chiropractic researcher usually associates with an accredited chiropractic college, hospital, clinic, health and welfare organization, or private industry.


## PREVENTIVE HEALTH CARE

Americans lag far behind many countries of the world in physical fitness. Space age developments have encouraged a life-style of minimal physical effort. Nature, however, is not wasteful. What is not used, degenerates. Our physical fitness is no exception.

Since its development, the chiropractic profession has offered national and community leadership in encouraging parents and teachers to support physical fitness programs in schools. In homes, youngsters must be encouraged to develop good fitness and health habits at an early age. Fitness is a family affair.

When biomechanics are disturbed through stress and strain, distortion results because of the interrelationship of our structural and functional systems. Posture not only has a direct bearing on comfort and work efficiency; it is also a factor which determines resistance to disease and disability.

Chiropractic is attentive to the importance of nerve integrity and body mechanics for good health. The doctor of chiropractic is concerned with the effects and prevention of spinal defects affecting physical fitness. He or she is trained to treat many health problems and this treatment is aimed at maintaining mechanical integrity by correcting spinal and extraspinal defects and postural distortions.

To assure health, our bodies must be free from structural distortions and must operate at peak efficiency. Any activity in which the structure of the human frame is thrown out of normal balance can cause distortion of the spine, which not only supports the weight of the entire body above the pelvis but also protects the spinal cord.

As early as 1930, the White House Conference on Child Health recognized the importance of spinal integrity and body mechanics in relation to health. Correct posture is essential to proper development, balance, coordination, rhythm, and timing. There is an undisputed relationship between good posture and good health.

A spinal injury or defect may not have dramatic effects. It may occur subtly and grow worse with time. Unless trained in the health sciences, most people do not usually recognize subtle health problems; they learn instead to adapt and suffer in silence. As a result, many spinal defects are unknown until the problem grows more serious and pain is felt. To add to the mystery, symptoms often occur in a part of the body not ordinarily associated with the spine. For this reason, chiropractic care is attentive to the cause.

It is unfortunate that the subluxation, and its attendant soft-tissue trauma, is one of the most commonly overlooked diagnoses within the healing arts. Mechanical disorders and their functional alterations are probably the most common human ills today. This is not unusual when we consider the body's response to gravity is a constant strain in the upright posture. Such stress must have a negative effect on the healing powers of our nature. We should be ever mindful that the musculoskeletal system comprises more than 60 percent of our body's total mass; this 60 percent is often overlooked within the healing arts.

## NUTRITIONAL AND EXERCISE CONSIDERATIONS

In addition to the correction of biomechanical faults, the development of good posture habits, and the necessity for regular exercise, nutrition plays an important role in maintaining health. Nourishing food that builds bone and muscle and maintains nerve and blood integrity is essential to good health.

Too often in our society, a well-balanced diet has been replaced by manufactured sweets, snack foods, and TV dinners. Toxic substances in these foods weaken our natural resistance.

Although all natural foods contain the nutrients necessary for their metabolism, they seldom retain their original vitamins when they reach the table. While caloric values and the quantity and quality of protein, carbohydrate, and fat are relatively unchanged, at least six vitamins can be lost or partly destroyed by steaming, frying, roasting, boiling, freezing, or drying. Industrialized food processing often results in a deficiency of vitamins and elements necessary for metabolism. Many trace elements which were once plentiful in American soil have been grossly depleted through the use of commercial fertilizers.

While meat is a common source of protein, it must be kept in mind that meat is commonly infused with an array of antibiotics, artificial sex hormones, and a round of additives designed to preserve, age, cure, and tenderize. Fruits and vegetables commonly purchased at the corner supermarket contain a degree of pesticide residue. Without question, many common food processing techniques and additives have a nefarious effect upon our natural resistance and recuperative powers.

Maintaining cellular and biochemical balance by supplying proper nutrients is the purpose of nutrition and a primary basis of good health. Yet, a number of authorities claim that Americans are the most overfed and undernourished people in the world. Dietary management under chiropractic care is thus often necessary to see that the diet provides balanced meals made up of proteins, carbohydrates, and fats, and the nutrients necessary for proper metabolism. Nutrition is an important part of the curriculum at each accredited chiropractic college.

## HOSPITAL PRACTICE

Although many doctors of chiropractic are engaged in private practice, many can be found in partnerships, group practices, outpatient clinics, and health care centers.

A recent trend is for the chiropractor to branch out into HMO organizations, PPO organizations, state planning and regulatory bodies, as well as integrating into hospital settings. Many hospital staffs now consist of psychologists, dentists, podiatrists, and as of this writing, there are approximately 12 hospitals which have granted chiropractors limited co-admitting privileges. Many health care authorities predict that the outcomes of the chiropractic involvement by the various hospitals currently granting staff privileges will determine the future for increased hospital participation.

There is no question that as chiropractic demonstrates its effective, conservative management in various ailments under hospital supervision, there will be an increased demand for chiropractic by both the patients and the medical community.

The future of chiropractors as hospital staff physicians cannot be explored within the context of this career book, but the future of chiropractic will remain inextricably related to ongoing research and carefully supervised clinical trials. The hospital environment will undoubtedly help to erase any interdisciplinary antagonism which had been evident in the past. Team-oriented physicians of all disciplines will be the wave of the new health care practitioner of tomorrow.

## MENTAL HEALTH

Professor William James of Harvard, the father of American psychology, contended that, while emotional disturbances can cause structural and functional disorders, structural and functional disorders can also cause emotional disturbances. Thus, the structural-neurological approach of chiropractic may often benefit the diagnosis and treatment of associated behavioral disorders. The ACA Council on Mental Health continues to monitor the scientific literature to fortify increasing evidence of chiropractic's somato-psychic approach to mental health.


## PRENATAL AND POSTNATAL CARE

During pregnancy there is a natural change within the pel-vic structures, along with an accompanying change in weight distribution. Health disorders such as headaches, backaches, leg pains, and lower-extremity circulatory disturbances may often be attributed solely to the strain upon the musculo-skeletal system. In association with regular obstetrical care, periodic chiropractic spinal checks and adjustments throughout the course of pregnancy have shown excellent clinical results in either reducing or eliminating such disor-ders, as well as in easing the labor or delivery.

The strain of delivery, coupled with the disproportionate weight of the child's head upon yet-to-be-fully-developed neck structures, may result in injury to the child's upper cer-vical vertebrae and related soft tissues. Chiropractors rec-ommend a spinal examination of the child as soon as possible after birth so that proper corrections can be made if problems exist. Empirical results have shown that chiroprac-tic pediatric examination and care during the postnatal period has positive influence on reducing the possibility of colic, digestive sensitivities, allergies, and other common dysfunctions in the newborn.

Since it is impossible to restrain a normal child from par-ticipating in the numerous activities that may cause stress and strain, the correction of faulty body mechanics during the early stages of development is important. Active children are particularly prone to spinal subluxation because they are energetic, impatient, and have an innocent disregard for cau-tion. Spinal disorders often are the result of twists, sudden turns, awkward lifts and postural positions, and jolts to the body during ordinary activity. If not corrected, spinal problems may lead to interference with normal function and body mechanics causing or contributing to severe illness.

While chiropractors emphasize the importance of the correction of spinal and extraspinal mechanical lesions, no practitioner believes that these are the sole causes of disease. However, clinical chiropractic has repeatedly shown that spinal problems are a contributing or inducing factor involved in many more dysfunctions than is commonly realized. When combined with poor nutrition, poor physical fitness and posture, environmental pollutants, physical and emotional stress, bacteria, viruses, rickettsia, molds, yeasts, worms, trauma, and other debilitating factors, such mechanical lesions become a vital consideration.

## RELIEF OF PAIN

In matters of health, a warning signal, such as pain, matters a great deal. Pain is nature's alarm that tells us that our body is not functioning properly—that something serious may be wrong with our health. It is just as foolhardy simply to kill the pain with a pill or injection as it would be to silence a fire alarm without seeking its cause. To affect proper care, the cause must be treated—not just the symptom. In many cases, pain may occur in our body in a location different from the source of the trouble.

Headaches are the most common complaint encountered in patients by practitioners of the healing arts. A common cause of headaches is disorders originating from spinal problems in the neck. It is important that such mechanical lesions be recognized by a trained chiropractic physician. Unfortunately, headaches are too often offered a generalized diagnosis such as sinus trouble, migraine, cluster headaches, and so on. Because chiropractic care is attentive to the biomechanics and neurocirculatory implications involved, headache sufferers have frequently found relief under chiropractic care.

The second most common complaint is that of backache. Here again, lumbago, sacroiliac strains, and disc injuries are of a musculoskeletal nature with neurologic overtones. It is important that the cause be recognized and cared for before permanent damage is done. Because chiropractic care recognizes the structural/functional relationships involved, the profession has earned a respected reputation in handling cases of both acute and chronic spinal pain.

## SPORTS INJURIES

Because of chiropractic's emphasis upon structural/ functional relationships in health and disease processes, it is logical that there is much attention within the profession given to therapeutic kinesiology—the study of human movement. For many years, the American Chiropractic Association has encouraged development of the Council on Sports Injuries. The purpose of the council is to seek improvement in the areas of prevention and correction of health problems in sports and recreational activities. Because of chiropractic input, counsel, and ingenuity, several contributions have been made in regard to protective gear in contact sports, athletic health maintenance, therapy, and enhanced rehabilitation after injury.

While chiropractic contributions in this area have been made for many years, the public press has brought attention to the profession's unique approach. Much publicity surrounding chiropractic care with Olympic athletes of several countries has been carried by the wire services and sports magazines before and during recent Olympic games.

Because of their witness to demonstrated chiropractic efficiency in the care, treatment, and prevention of athletic injuries, several outstanding athletes have entered the chiropractic profession.

## INSURANCE CASES

Many Americans carry health and accident insurance or other third-party payment plans that cover all or part of their costs for health care services. There are many types of insurance. Most pay for chiropractic services; a few do not. Third-party payment for chiropractic care is becoming more popular each year and is expected to receive full coverage in the future. Those programs operated through state and federal agencies for special groups are also expected to increase. Some are designed to help veterans and servicemen and their dependents, some for the aged and the indigent.

## WOMEN IN CHIROPRACTIC

Chiropractic welcomes women to the profession and admits them to all accredited chiropractic colleges. Although more than 10 percent of the doctors of chiropractic are presently women, there is great need for more women doctors. This percentage is higher than for medicine, dentistry, optometry and law, and strikingly illustrates the unusual advantages accruing to women in this profession.

A study of accredited chiropractic colleges for the period

1979–1982 revealed an increase in enrollment of more than 24 percent in female students, from 7,948 to 9,887. While the number of males grew by over 16 percent, from 6,568 to 7,658, their proportion of the total enrollees decreased from 82.63 percent to 77.46 percent, whereas the number of enrolled women went from 1,380 to 2,229, an increase of over 61 percent. Similarly, the proportion of women increased from 17.37 percent to 22.54 percent. The total number of female graduates has gone from 1,557 to 2,388, an increase of over 53 percent. Women represented 12.46 percent of 1979 graduates and 18.13 percent of 1982 graduates.

When compared with the professions of dentistry, medicine, and law, it is apparent that chiropractic colleges are following the same trend of enrolling more women and bestowing more degrees upon women.

## CHIROPRACTIC IN FOREIGN LANDS

The practice of chiropractic is officially regulated in nine of the provinces of Canada, in Australia, New Zealand, Switzerland, and West Germany. It is acknowledged and accepted in Belgium, Bolivia, Denmark, France, Great Britain, Italy, Japan, the Netherlands, Norway, Peru, South Africa, Sweden, Venezuela, and Zimbabwe, but not to the extent that it is in officially regulated countries.

## CHIROPRACTIC MISSIONARIES

The Christian Chiropractors Association places world missions at the heart of its program. Presently sponsoring a number of different missions, the group looks forward to enlarging the range of its missions in the future. At the present time, the association is represented by chiropractic missionaries in Indonesia, Peru, Quebec, Bolivia, Ethiopia, Monaco, Israel, Hong Kong, Mexico, and the United States.

## PROFESSIONAL AND ECONOMIC REWARDS

A career in chiropractic offers real, lasting satisfaction and rewarding income. In addition, doctors of chiropractic are their own managers. They establish their own hours and work habits. The chiropractic physician enjoys the advantages of a profession that is well established; one that ranks high in prestige and service, does not limit opportunity, income, or challenge; and yet offers opportunities of security and community leadership. Chiropractic offers opportunity to serve and receive in abundance.

*Independence.* Doctors of chiropractic are their own employers. If they enter independent private practice, they have a wide choice of locations in any type of community they desire: in city, town, or rural area. They may have their office in a building downtown or in a residential area. They alone determine the hours they work. They are able to arrange their hours by appointment to suit their convenience. They determine when they will take their vacations and their days off.

*Prestige.* Doctors of chiropractic enjoy the respect of their patients and community. They earn the gratitude of all for fulfilling an honorable and needed function—that of maintaining the health and welfare of the people. They are looked up to as leaders, and as such have the opportunity to make many friends and to achieve social and civic prominence. Chiropractic office hours allow ample time to enjoy a full schedule of social, business, and professional activities. And the personal contacts made professionally and socially often enable D.C.'s to reach positions of leadership.

*Good Income.* The chiropractic profession is not interested in attracting students who are solely interested in financial gain. Rather, chiropractic wants earnest young men and women who will find gratification in contributing to human betterment. However, earning power should certainly be taken into account when determining a career. The earning potential of a doctor of chiropractic is good—as good as and often better than other professions. An ACA membership survey of 1982 indicated an annual gross income median among practitioners of $107,000 per year, with a net of $50,500.

As in other professions, financial success depends upon many factors: the individual characteristics of the practitioner, the doctor's ability to apply her or his knowledge, the doctor's personality, the location of practice, and local economic conditions. Statistics show, however, that professional people on the whole, regardless of personal circumstances, enjoy a greater degree of security and higher income than any other group.

## CHIROPRACTIC PARAPROFESSIONALS

A certified chiropractic assistant may be defined as an individual who has received advanced education in chiropractic philosophy, terminology, various diagnostic procedures, anatomy and physiology, clinical laboratory, ethics and jurisprudence, radiological technology, adjunctive therapy, and basic office procedures. Such individuals are professional aides to the doctor of chiropractic, under whose direct guidance and supervision they perform various duties involving basic office responsibilities and the preparation, management, and care of patients, including much instruction.

There are presently few national licensing provisions for chiropractic assistants. Florida, Illinois, Oklahoma, and Maryland have enacted legislation, and other states are now considering some manner of licensure.

Several chiropractic and liberal arts colleges have given recognition to and developed an educational curriculum for this special training. These programs were initiated to meet the needs and responsibilities of the chiropractic physician as the primary health care provider.

Plans are presently being developed within chiropractic post-graduate education to encourage greater use of chiropractic assistants to increase professional productivity. State and national chiropractic organizations, in conjunction with chiropractic colleges, are developing plans to pass legislation which would establish a nationwide accredited chiropractic assistant program. By the summer of 1982, there were approximately 41,000 chiropractic assistants employed nationwide.

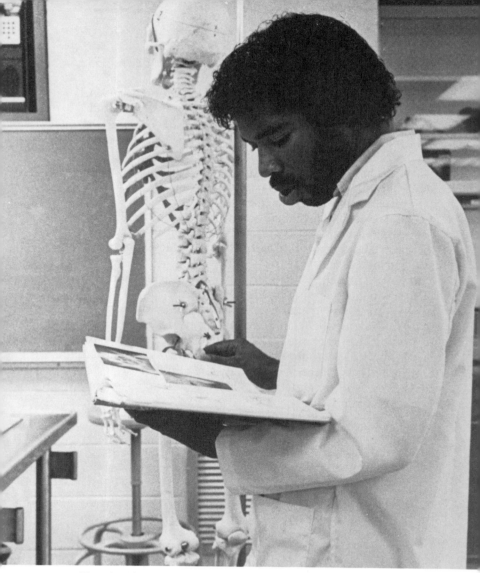

The educational preparation of a doctor of chiropractic is demanding but rewarding. Special attention to the musculoskeletal and nervous system is what is unique in chiropractic education. The vertebral subluxation complex is currently being investigated and researched in most chiropractic institutions.

**CHAPTER 5**

# EDUCATIONAL PREPARATION

By the early 1980s, nine chiropractic colleges in the United States had become fully accredited and six colleges had been granted Recognized Candidate for Accreditation (RCA) status with the Council on Chiropractic Education (CCE), an autonomous corporation sponsored by the American Chiropractic Association, the International Chiropractors Association, and the Federation of Chiropractic Licensing Boards. All but a few chiropractic licensing boards require that their applicants be graduates of a college with CCE status.

Chiropractic colleges require a minimum of four academic years of professional resident study, including clinical experience under strict supervision, preceded by a minimum of two years of college work with a prescribed content. The first two years of professional study emphasize life sciences, health sciences, and clinical disciplines. The remaining two years emphasize practical or clinical studies dealing with the diagnosis and treatment of disease, with approximately half the time spent in college clinics.

## THE COUNCIL ON CHIROPRACTIC EDUCATION (CCE)

The CCE and its Commission on Accreditation are recognized by the U.S. Department of Education as the sole reliable authority on the quality of training offered by chiropractic colleges.

To assure that high educational standards are maintained, the CCE has established a Commission on Accreditation. Certain requirements must be met before a chiropractic college is considered for evaluation. First, requirements for a standard curriculum must be met. Second, prescriptions are set by the CCE for faculty qualifications, faculty-student ratios, library holdings, and physical plant, as well as for school governance, administration, and financial stability. Third, a student entrance requirement of a minimum of two years of college work with a prescribed science content must be met.

The CCE is also recognized by the Council on Postsecondary Accreditation (COPA) for programs leading to the Doctor of Chiropractic degree. COPA, a private, nonprofit educational association, evaluates and recognizes responsible accrediting agencies in the United States. In addition, the CEE is a member of the Council of Specialized Accrediting Agencies (CSAA), an autonomous, nongovernmental accreditation agency. CSAA fosters the maintenance of high standards within the wide spectrum of postsecondary education.

## PREPROFESSIONAL EDUCATION

All candidates to a chiropractic college must furnish proof of having acquired at least two years (or sixty acceptable semester hours) of studies leading to a baccalaureate degree in the arts and sciences, including laboratory courses in biology and chemistry. No more than twenty semester hours of a candidate's preprofessional education may be acquired through CLEP examinations.

## PROFESSIONAL EDUCATION

*Purpose.* The purpose of the curriculum is to provide the means for giving a student a thorough understanding of the structure and function of the human organism in health and disease. A well-balanced presentation gives the student an understanding of the essential features of the life processes: digestion, excretion, physical and mental growth, nutrition, metabolism, energy, nervous control, the significance of development defects, behavior, and other elements which are fundamental to the understanding of pathological conditions. This understanding makes it possible for students to identify deviations from the normal and provides the essential knowledge required for diagnosis, prognosis, and treatment.

*Length and Sequence of Course.* The curriculum is presented over a minimum period of eight semesters or the equivalent, for a total of not less than 4,200 hours. The course is presented in a sequence of subjects to insure proper prerequisites.

*Offerings.* The offerings include the following disciplines: human anatomy; biochemistry; physiology; microbiology; pathology; public health; physical, clinical, and laboratory diagnosis; gynecology; obstetrics; pediatrics; geriatrics; dermatology; otolaryngology; roentgenology; psychology; dietetics; orthopedics; physical therapy; first aid and emergency procedures; spinal analysis; principles and practice of chiropractic; adjustive technique; research methods and procedure; and other appropriate subjects. Such courses are taught in sufficient depth to fulfill the concept of the chiropractic physician as set forth within the educational standards of the Council on Chiropractic Education.

The above standards of the CCE have been adopted by the Federation of Chiropractic Licensing Boards (FCLB). The FCLB has recommended to the various state licensing boards that a rule of law be adopted, either by statute or by administrative regulation, where it will be provided that:

> All applicants for licensure who matriculate in a chiropractic college after October 1, 1975, must present evidence of having graduated from a chiropractic college having status with the Commission on Accreditation of the Council on Chiropractic Education, or its successor, or from a chiropractic college which meets equivalent standards thereof.

As of 1984, licensing jurisdictions of thirty-nine states or territories have sent formal letters indicating statutory or administrative code changes reflecting Federation policy, or are in various stages of procedure leading to the adoption of changes in licensing reflecting Federation policy.


## PERSONAL ATTRIBUTES

Personal qualifications should include above-average mental ability, ability to manage time and work independently, a strong desire to serve the sick, ability to maintain high ethical and professional standards, understanding, empathy, tact, patience, adaptability, ability to inspire confidence and respect, high moral character and integrity, manual skill and dexterity, and a keen sense of observation.

## SELECTING A CHIROPRACTIC COLLEGE

The most important decision for the prospective student is the selection of a college. The thoroughness of your training will determine the success or failure of your entire career. Chiropractic has evolved from the pioneer stage into a modern profession with high standards of education similar to those of other professions.

The CCE periodically inspects and issues a list of approved colleges. These colleges meet the license requirements of various states in the United States and of most of the provinces of Canada. There are still a few unapproved schools whose courses, in the opinion of the CCE, are not of the same grade of excellence as those of the approved colleges. However, all approved chiropractic colleges offer a comprehensive course of study which prepares the student to pass licensing examinations and perform competently in the profession.

Students should choose a college as early in their pre-professional careers as possible. This will permit them to take the exact courses needed to succeed in chiropractic college. Although chances of admittance are high, colleges are becoming more and more selective each year. To increase chances of acceptance, students should apply to two or three colleges.

Although most students attend chiropractic colleges in the United States, students may apply to foreign colleges. These colleges are located in English-speaking countries, so there is no language barrier. However, travel expenses and the lack of fellowships and scholarships may be a hindrance to some prospective students.

College officials will weigh all applications against a number of factors that includes grades in high school and in the two or more years of prechiropractic college training, and the extracurricular activities which show evidence of the student's ability to get along with others.

International students must meet the same preprofessional academic criteria as American students. Furthermore, international students must have valid documents of admission to the United States. If any questions arise about the American equivalency of the student's international training, it is the responsibility of the student to obtain a letter of explanation and approval from the CCE.

Some students can obtain advanced standing in individual cases. A student needs to check carefully with the chosen college for its rules and regulations. Students requesting advanced standing are usually required to prove that the content of courses they have already completed is equivalent to those of the college where they seek advanced standing. If the school from which the student wishes to transfer credits is not accredited by the CCE, courses are accepted only on a provisional basis. Advanced standing for courses taken at an accredited liberal arts college is often granted for hours above the sixty semester hour prerequisite.

## THE PERSONAL INTERVIEW

Students can expect a personal interview even if their grades are high and they have the best references, since all students are in competition for a place in an entering class. Although the interviewer will attempt to put the student at ease, the prospective applicant should think about some of the questions that the interviewer might ask and outline what might be said. Sample questions are: Why do you want to be a doctor of chiropractic? How much contact have you had with chiropractic? What do you know about the field? Are you interested in science? Do you make friends easily? How do you feel about working around sick people?

During an interview, students should relax and answer the questions as honestly as they can. They should not attempt to put on a false front. They should base their answers on the relevance of the questions to their future careers. The interviewer should be shown that the student has a sincere interest in chiropractic as demonstrated by her or his activities.

## ACCREDITED AND RECOGNIZED
## CANDIDATE COLLEGES

As of 1987, the following colleges have achieved accredited status or are recognized as candidates for accreditation (RCA). Recognized candidates for accreditation are identified by an asterisk (*).

CLEVELAND CHIROPRACTIC COLLEGE
6401 Rockhill Road
Kansas City, MO    64131

CLEVELAND CHIROPRACTIC COLLEGE
590 N. Vermont Avenue
Los Angeles, CA    90004

LIFE CHIROPRACTIC COLLEGE
1269 Barclay Circle
Marietta, GA    30060

LIFE CHIROPRACTIC COLLEGE-WEST
2005 Via Barrett, Box 367
San Lorenzo, CA    94580

LOGAN COLLEGE OF CHIROPRACTIC
P. O. Box 100, 1851 Schoettler Road
Chesterfield, MO    63017

LOS ANGELES COLLEGE OF CHIROPRACTIC
P. O. Box 1166, 16200 E. Amber Valley Drive
Whittier, CA    90609

NATIONAL COLLEGE OF CHIROPRACTIC
200 E. Roosevelt Road
Lombard, IL    60148

NEW YORK CHIROPRACTIC COLLEGE
P. O. Box 167
Glen Head, NY    11545

NORTHWESTERN COLLEGE OF CHIROPRACTIC
2501 W. 84th Street
Bloomington, MN    55431

PALMER COLLEGE OF CHIROPRACTIC
1000 Brady Street
Davenport, IA    52803

PALMER COLLEGE OF CHIROPRACTIC-WEST
1095 Dunford Way
Sunnyvale, CA    94087

PARKER COLLEGE OF CHIROPRACTIC*
300 E. Irving Blvd., P.O. Box 157444
Irving, TX    75060

TEXAS CHIROPRACTIC COLLEGE
5912 Spencer Highway
Pasadena, TX    77505

WESTERN STATES CHIROPRACTIC COLLEGE
2900 N.E. 132nd Avenue
Portland, OR    97230

*CCE ACCREDITED COLLEGES (Foreign)*

CANADIAN    MEMORIAL    CHIROPRACTIC    COLLEGE
(CCE/Canada)
1900 Bayview Avenue
Toronto, Ontario, Canada    M4G 3E6

PHILLIP INSTITUTE OF TECHNOLOGY (CCE/Australasia)
Plenty Road, Bundoora
Victoria, 3083, Australia

RCA status indicates that the institution is in compliance with the basic eligibility requirements for accreditation through self-study and the consultative assistance of the Commission on Accreditation of The Council on Chiropractic Education. Such status is not the same as accreditation, however, nor does it assure eventual accreditation.

Currently, one college is a CCE-affiliate member without status:

ANGLO-EUROPEAN COLLEGE OF CHIROPRACTIC
13-15 Parkwood Road
Bournemouth, England    BH5 2DF


## PROFILE OF A TYPICAL CHIROPRACTIC STUDENT

The typical student is male (17.8 percent female) and 24 years of age. About half of the students are married and have an average of one child. This typical student is a United States citizen (4.7 percent foreign).

Prior to entering chiropractic college, the student attended an accredited college and/or university for over 2.9 years, during which time he or she completed 60 semester hours of college credit, including a prescribed curriculum of biologic and physical science courses. College records indicate 13 percent entered with associate degrees, 35 percent with bachelor's degrees, 4 percent with Ph.D. degrees, and 0.4 percent held other degrees.

The student was a chiropractic patient (64.1 percent) and received information on chiropractic as a career from a doctor of chiropractic (65.5 percent). There is about a fifty-fifty chance that after graduation the new chiropractor will practice in a community of over 50,000 population.


## COST OF CHIROPRACTIC EDUCATION

In higher education generally, and in professional education particularly, the cost to the student is far less than the total educational cost involved. In chiropractic colleges, this difference is subsidized by the profession and by contributions from friends. The American Chiropractic Association allocates a substantial portion of its dues to both education and research. Specific information on costs to the student will be found in the annual college catalog of each institution.

It is certain that the student's expenses will be higher than anticipated. A good budget should incorporate some money for unexpected items.

In general, a student today can expect tuition to run approximately $2,000 a semester, plus $250 for miscellaneous fees and required books. See Table 1. Living expenses are not included in these estimates. Only a few chiropractic colleges have dormitories or apartments available to students. Living costs vary a great deal according to the tastes of the individual student. For a nine-month school year, living expenses are estimated at about $5,500 for a single student living in a room in a private home or shared apartment. This figure does not include clothes, entertainment, or travel.

When students enter clinical studies they will be required to purchase basic diagnostic instruments such as stethoscope, otoscope, and a blood measuring apparatus (sphygmomanometer). New, these items cost approximately $400 to $600. Slightly used books and diagnostic equipment can often be purchased at a greatly reduced price.

## TABLE 1. APPROXIMATE SEMESTER TUITION

| Chiropractic College | Basic Tuition* | Books and Equipment Fees, Avg.* | Per Academic Calendar |
|---|---|---|---|
| Cleveland (Kansas City) | $2585 | $300 | Trimester |
| Cleveland (Los Angeles) | 2800 | 400 | Trimester |
| Life | 1825 | 150 | Quarter |
| Life-West | 2000 | 200 | Quarter |
| Logan | 2625 | 350 | Trimester |
| Los Angeles | 2860 | 275 | Trimester |
| National | 2764 | 300 | Trimester |
| New York | 2650 | 350 | Trimester |
| Northwestern | 2800 | 325 | Trimester |
| Palmer | 1715 | 185 | Quarter |
| Palmer-West | 1990 | 225 | Quarter |
| Parker | 2400 | 250 | Trimester |
| Pasadena | 1800 | 160 | Trimester |
| Texas | 2600 | 170 | Trimester |
| Western States | 2250 | 350 | Quarter |

*Foreign CCE Accredited Colleges By Reciprocal Agreement*

| | | | |
|---|---|---|---|
| Canadian Memorial | 6000 | 790 | Academic Year |
| | 7500 (foreign) | | |
| Phillip Institute of Technology | Govt. funded | 175 | Academic Year |

*Affiliate College (Foreign)*

| | | | |
|---|---|---|---|
| Anglo-European | 4700 | 400 | Academic Year |

*Figures as of January 1987

## STUDENT SCHOLARSHIPS

Various types of scholarships are available at all chiropractic colleges. The sources or the donors of the scholarship vary as does the amount of each scholarship. State funds may also be available. Many states have commissions established for disbursement of funds to public and private nonprofit institutions for financial aid to eligible students.

There are also several privately funded scholarships offered each year on a national basis; e.g., through the Colonel Harland B. Sanders Trust, the Springwall Trust, the Vitaminerals Scholarship Fund, state chiropractic associations, auxiliary organizations, fraternal organizations, etc. In addition, each college has its private scholarship programs. Eligibility requirements are set by the sponsor of the scholarship. Generally, scholarships are awarded on the basis of academic achievement and financial need. For further information, contact the Financial Aid Office of the college of your choice.

## STUDENT FINANCIAL AID

In addition to scholarships, several forms of financial aid via grants, loans, and study-work programs are available at chiropractic colleges. These opportunities have become increasingly important as the costs of health education increase.

All applicants for financial aid must be citizens of the United States, and applications for financial aid can only be made by those students who have been accepted by a specific college and have submitted the required entrance deposits.

# CHIROPRATIC COLLEGE CAMPUSES

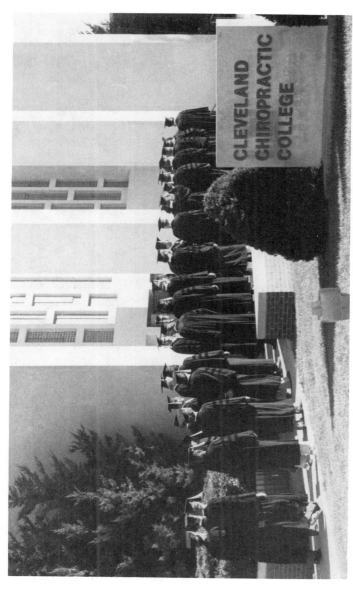

**CLEVELAND CHIROPRACTIC COLLEGE (1922)**
6401 Rockhill Road
Kansas City, MO 64131

(816) 333-8230

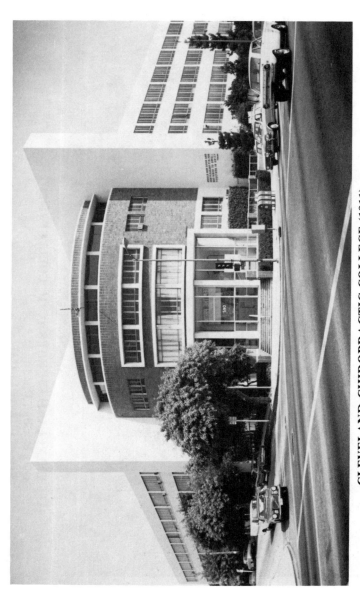

**CLEVELAND CHIROPRACTIC COLLEGE (1911)**
590 N. Vermont Avenue
Los Angeles, CA 90004

(213) 660-6166

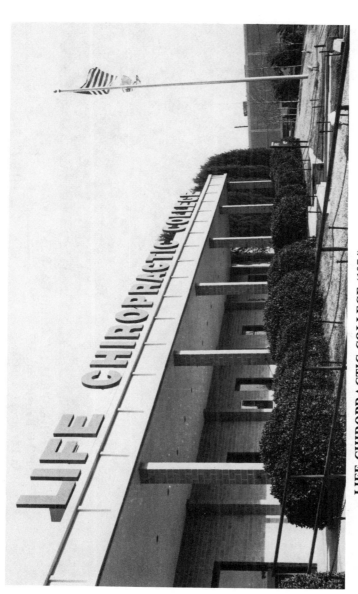

**LIFE CHIROPRACTIC COLLEGE (1974)**
1269 Barclay Circle
Marietta, GA 30060

(404) 424-0554

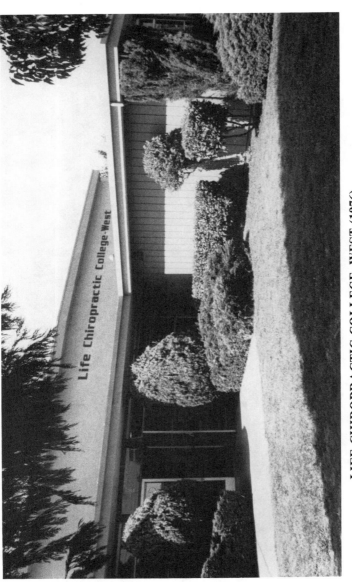

**LIFE CHIROPRACTIC COLLEGE–WEST (1976)**
2005 Via Barrett, Box 367
San Lorenzo, CA 94580

(415) 276-9013

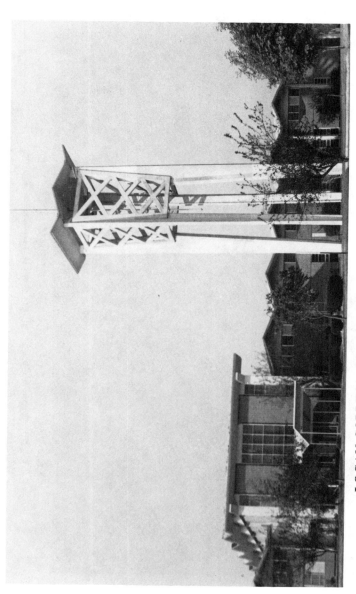

**LOGAN COLLEGE OF CHIROPRACTIC (1935)**
P.O. Box 100, 1851 Schoettler Road
Chesterfield, MO 63017

(314) 227-2100

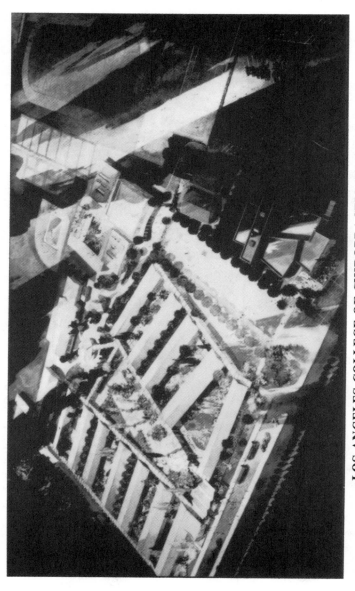

**LOS ANGELES COLLEGE OF CHIROPRACTIC (1911)**
P.O. Box 1166, 16200 E. Amber Valley Drive
Whittier, CA 90609-1166

(213) 947-8755

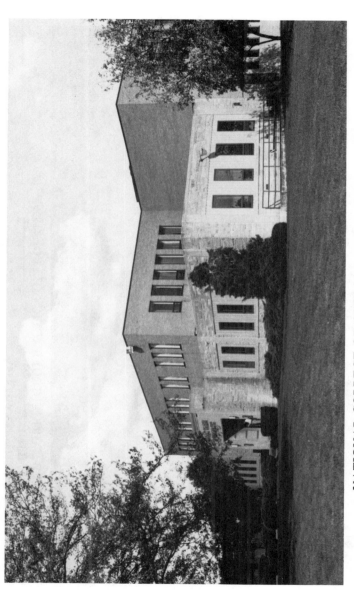

**NATIONAL COLLEGE OF CHIROPRACTIC (1906)**

200 E. Roosevelt Road

Lombard, IL 60148

(312) 629-2000

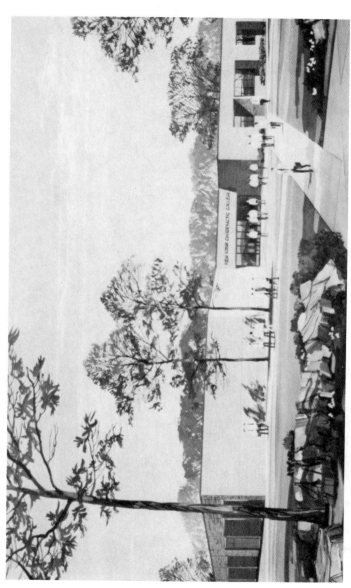

**NEW YORK CHIROPRACTIC COLLEGE (1919)**
P.O. Box 167
Glen Head, NY 11545

(516) 626-2700

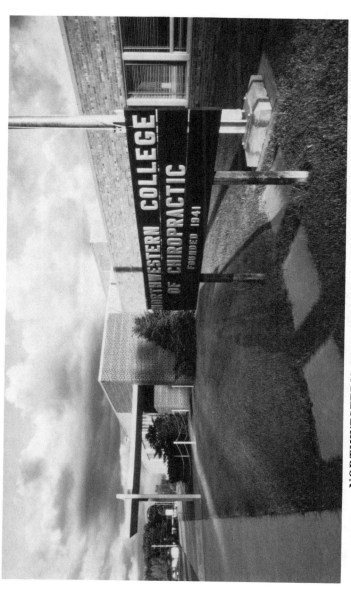

**NORTHWESTERN COLLEGE OF CHIROPRACTIC (1941)**
2501 W. 84th Street
Bloomington, MN 55431

(612) 888-4777

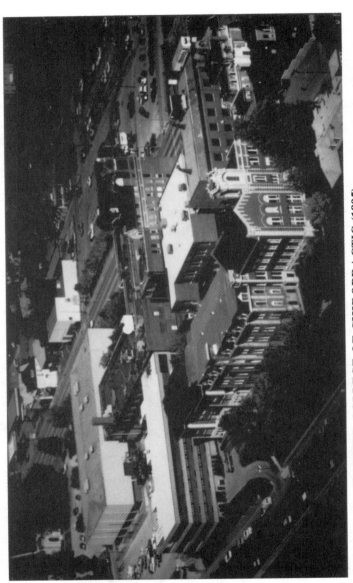

**PALMER COLLEGE OF CHIROPRACTIC (1895)**
1000 Brady Street
Davenport, IA 52803

(319) 326-9600

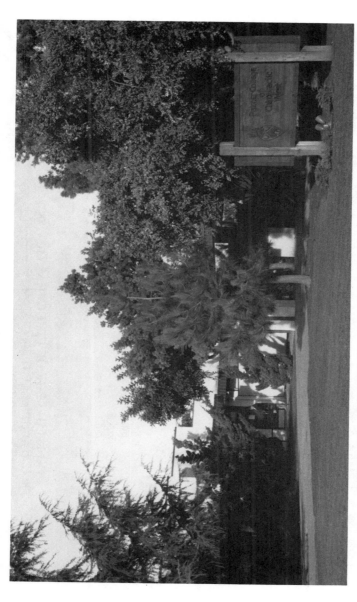

**PALMER COLLEGE OF CHIROPRACTIC–WEST (1978)**
1095 Dunford Way
Sunnyvale, CA 94087

(408) 244-8907

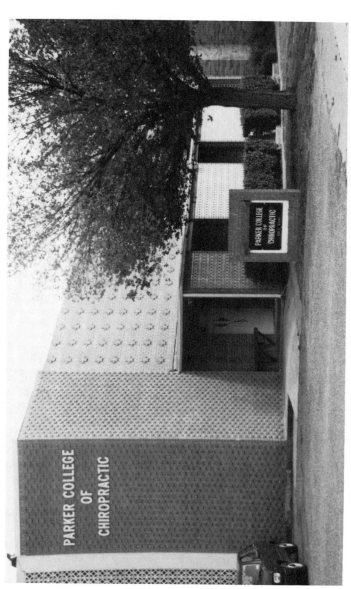

**PARKER COLLEGE OF CHIROPRACTIC (1982)**
300 E. Irving Blvd., P.O. Box 157444
Irving, TX 75060-3038

(214) 438-6932

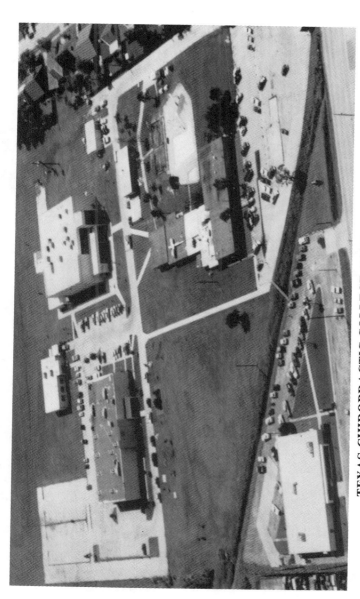

**TEXAS CHIROPRACTIC COLLEGE (1908)**
5912 Spencer Highway
Pasadena, TX 77505

(713) 487-1170

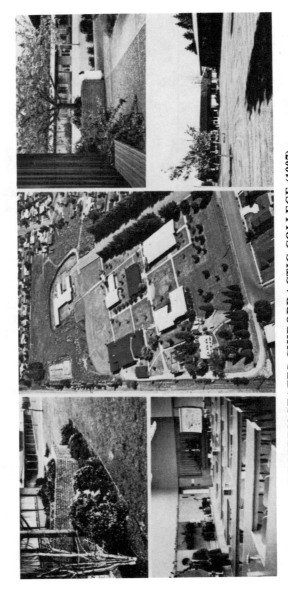

**WESTERN STATES CHIROPRACTIC COLLEGE** (1907)
2900 N.E. 132nd Avenue
Portland, OR 97230-3099

(503) 256-3180

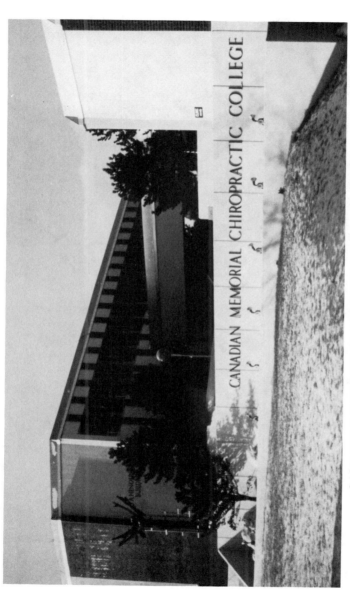

**CANADIAN MEMORIAL CHIROPRACTIC COLLEGE**
1900 Bayview Avenue
Toronto, Ontario, Canada M4G 3E6          (416) 482-2340

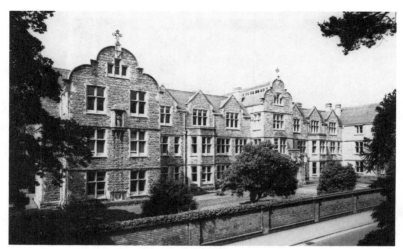

**ANGLO-EUROPEAN COLLEGE OF CHIROPRACTIC**
13-15 Parkwood Road
Bournemouth, England, BH5 2DF

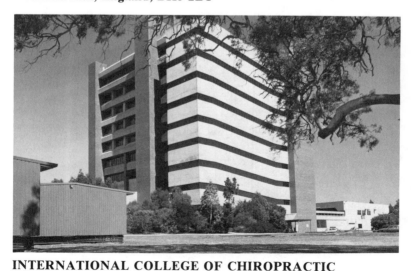

**INTERNATIONAL COLLEGE OF CHIROPRACTIC**
School of Chiropractic
Phillip Institute of Technology
P.O. Box 96, Bundoora, Victoria, 3083, Australia   (03) 468-2200

As financial aid funds must be distributed among those students actually enrolled, financial aid can only be awarded to those students who have reserved a position within the next term. After the entrance deposit has been received and a position has been held within classes, the necessary application forms will be forwarded to the student. This usually includes a financial need analysis form that must be completed.

Prospective students should keep in mind that chiropractic colleges seek to aid students with limited financial resources the best they can. However, as the amount of aid available is limited, it should be assumed that students will use their own resources (including Pell Grants and family contributions) to the fullest extent prior to applying for other forms of assistance. Only after these resources have been exhausted will a college be able to offer further assistance with funds over which it is custodian.

## STUDENT GRANTS

*Pell Grant (PG).* For students who are eligible, this should be the *first* form of financial aid investigated. Failure to apply for a Pell Grant may result in the loss of a substantial financial-aid resource. A Pell Grant is a gift of money available to eligible students who do not have a bachelor's degree. Awards typically range from $200 to $2,000. The student must be enrolled in the first two years of the chiropractic curriculum and not have earned more than 119 semester credits since graduation from high school. A Financial Aid Form (FAF) must be completed each year and sent to the College Scholarship Service (CSS) for processing, who will then at the college's request forward that information to the U.S. Department of Education for analysis to determine eligibility. This should be done before applications for student *loans* are made. Eligibility is determined within eight weeks after analysis of the student's and parents' income and assets. Notification is made via a Student Eligibility Report (SER). Half-time students are generally eligible to receive a proportionately reduced award. Pell Grant awards are disbursed to a student via the college or under an alternate disbursement system where the college certifies costs and the student sends the required forms and certificates to the federal government to receive the award.

*Supplemental Educational Opportunity Grant (SEOG).* This is a campus-based award of federal money given to colleges to be disbursed to needy eligible students who meet government regulations controlling this program. To qualify for these very limited funds, a student must be eligible for a Pell Grant and still have exceptional financial need as determined by the result of a financial need analysis. Forms to apply for this grant are available through the college's Financial Aid Office.

*Veteran Benefits.* Students who qualify can obtain benefits available under Chapter 34—Veteran's Educational Assistance and Chapter 31—Vocational Rehabilitation.


## STUDENT LOANS


*National Direct Student Loan (NDSL).* This type of loan is available only to continuing students with exceptional financial need after they have exhausted all other sources of financial aid. Applications for a NDSL may be made at the same time as students apply for other forms of campus-based aid such as a SEOG or CWS. Repayment begins six months after a student ceases to be enrolled at least half-time. The typical minimum payment is $30 per month and the maximum payment period is ten years. Interest is charged during the repayment period at a reduced rate (e.g., 5–6%/year) on the unpaid balance.

*Federally Insured and State Guaranteed Student Loans (FISL and GSL).* These loan programs enable undergraduate students to borrow up to $2,500 per academic year up to a maximum of $12,500. Graduate students may borrow up to $5,000 per academic year for their college experience to a cumulative amount of $25,000. Loans received at the undergraduate level are included in the $25,000 maximum unless they are paid back in full. Interested students should first attempt to seek a private lender such as a bank, credit union, etc., for a Guaranteed Student Loan. If a student is refused by a private lender in the student's area of legal residence, it is then usually possible to process such a loan directly through the state's Student Loan Program at a reasonable rate of interest (e.g., 9%). Schedules for loan payments on a GSL are established with graduates by the lending agency six months after graduation. At the time the loan papers are signed, the indebted student is informed of the exact amount of interest to be accrued and the number of interim months between graduation and the initiation of the payment schedule. Repayment usually begins six months following graduation or termination of at least half-time enrollment. The minimum monthly payment is $50, and the maximum payment period is ten years. The federal government pays the loan's interest until the repayment schedule is initiated. There is a prepaid finance charge for each loan and a 5% origination fee.

*Parent Loan for Undergraduate Students (PLUS).* The PLUS is an auxiliary student loan program designed to provide additional funds for educational expenses. It enables parents of students or independent undergraduates to borrow money on their own behalf directly from a private lender. It is possible to borrow up to $3,000 per academic year to a maximum of $15,000. The current interest rate is 12–14%. The loan amounts available via a PLUS program are in addition to the amounts that a student can borrow under a GSL program. However, a PLUS loan cannot exceed a student's cost of education. Repayment is made in monthly installments throughout and beyond the length of the student's education.

*Auxiliary Loans to Assist Students (ALAS).* These are nonsubsidized loans for undergraduate and graduate students that are similar to PLUS loans. Student borrowers may receive deferment of principal if they are full-time students, but they may be responsible for payment of the interest during the deferment period.

*Health Education Assistance Loan (HEAL).* This program is a federally insured loan program available to eligible chiropractic students. A student may borrow up to $12,500 a year, up to a maximum of $50,000 for the four-year curriculum. The amount of interest that may be charged to the borrower on the unpaid balance of the loan may not exceed the average bond-equivalent rate during the prior calendar quarter for 91-day Treasury Bills plus 3.5 percent and rounded to the next higher ⅛ of one percent (annual percentage rate). Currently, this amounts to 19.5 percent interest. Accrued interest may be compounded every six months by adding it to the principal of the loan. Repayment begins nine months after the borrower ceases to be a full-time student.

## STUDENT WORK-STUDY PROGRAMS

*College Work Study (CWS) Program.* This is a campus-based work program, jointly funded by the college and the federal government, that provides jobs on campus for students who work 5–20 hours each week at an hourly rate for undergraduate students determined by the position. Graduate students may be salaried. Time cards and personal production are carefully monitored. The institution provides available positions for students in areas of library, audiovisual aids, business office, admissions, clerical work, building maintenance, laboratory assistance, etc. As the support funds received from the Department of Education are limited, a student must demonstrate need as shown by a financial need analysis.

All questions concerning financial aid should be directed to the financial aid officer of the prospective chiropractic college.

## PART-TIME EMPLOYMENT

Many students find it necessary to supplement their means by part-time work while attending college. About half of the students attending approved chiropractic colleges engage in part-time work with or without the assistance of their schools. However, the curriculum demands the major portion of the student's time and energy. Therefore, it is not wise for a student to attempt to earn her or his entire college and living expenses, while at the same time trying to carry the required course of study.

## THE PROFESSIONAL DEGREE AND
## LICENSURE REQUIREMENTS

Upon acceptable completion of the college program, the degree of D.C. (Doctor of Chiropractic) is awarded. Candidates for graduation in all approved colleges must be at least 21 years of age. They must have completed the prescribed curriculum of the college and have complied with all its regulations. Persons registered as special students who already hold a doctorate in chiropractic cannot be candidates for a duplicate degree.

In all states, the District of Columbia, Puerto Rico, and in most Canadian provinces, there are specific laws governing the practice of chiropractic and prescribing requirements for chiropractic licensure. These jurisdictions have examining boards that are usually composed of chiropractic physicians and lay people. In a few states, there are composite boards of doctors of chiropractic and doctors of medicine. At the present time, most licensing jurisdictions recognize or utilize the certificate of the National Board of Chiropractic Examiners.

## ADMISSIONS

Regardless of lesser statutory requirements, all recognized chiropractic colleges require at least two years of 60 acceptable semester hours leading to a baccalaureate degree in the arts and sciences. Preprofessional credits must be earned at institutions listed in the *Education Directory—Higher Education* of the U.S. Department of Education. Applicants must be graduates of or eligible to return to the last institution attended, with an exception made where the applicant provides a letter of honorary dismissal from the last institution attended.

The preprofessional education that has been acquired must have an average of 2.25 on a 4.0 scale, with no less than a C grade in courses with laboratory in biology, chemistry, and physics. No more than 20 semester hours of a candidate's preprofessional education (in courses other than the natural, biological, and physical sciences) can have been acquired through CLEP examination or challenging courses. Matriculants must present a minimum of:

- *English or communicative skills*
  1 academic year, not less than 6 semester hours.
- *Psychology*
  ½ academic year, not less than 3 semester hours.
- *Social sciences or humanities*
  ½ academic year, not less than 3 semester hours.
- *Biological science (with related laboratory)*
  1 academic year, not less than 6 semester hours.
- *General or inorganic chemistry (with related laboratory)*
  1 academic year, not less than 6 semester hours.
- *Organic chemistry (with related laboratory)*
  1 academic year, not less than 6 semester hours.
- *Physics (with related laboratory)*
  1 academic year, not less than 6 semester hours.

## TRANSFER OF CREDITS

Transfer students must meet the admission requirements of the transferee institution at the time of the students' original matriculation. Such students must present the institution to be entered with a letter of recommendation from the transferor institution, and the students' transfer credits must be identifiable to the curriculum of the transferee institution. Credit for courses with a grade of 2 or better on a 4.0 scale is given. In addition, transferred credits cannot be used for double credit; i.e., they cannot be used to meet both prechiropractic and chiropractic requirements.

Where students have interrupted their chiropractic training for a period in excess of five years, credit is not allowed on re-enrollment or transfer for courses previously taken. Such student must also meet current admission requirements.

Recognized colleges may accept credits of transfer from institutions not having status with the Commission on Accreditation of the CCE. However, it is the responsibility of the accepting institution to inform such transfer students that they may, on the basis of those transfer credits, be ineligible for licensure in one or more states.

## ADVANCED STANDING

College equivalency credits may be accepted if an applicant has had certification of the credits by an approved institution of higher education. Advanced credits are based on official transcripts received directly from a chiropractic college acceptable to the Committee on Admissions of the college to be entered or from nonchiropractic but accredited institutions.

Applicants for admission to advanced standing are required to furnish evidence that: (1) they can meet the same entrance requirements as candidates for the first-year class; (2) courses equivalent in content and quality to those given in the admitting college in the year or years preceding that to which admission is desired have been satisfactorily completed; (3) the work was done in a chiropractic college acceptable to the Committee on Admissions of the college;

and (4) the candidate has a letter of recommendation from the dean of the college from which transfer is made.

Credits for work done in accredited colleges of liberal arts and sciences will be allowed only in nonclinical subjects. However, applicable credit may be granted to an applicant who has taken professional clinical work in an accredited medical or osteopathic college. No candidate will be accepted from such colleges if dishonorably dismissed.

For all students admitted to advanced standing, the college entered is required to have on file with the registrar (1) the same documents that are required for admission to the first-year class, (2) a certified transcript of work completed, and (3) a letter indicating honorable withdrawal from the college from which the transfer was made.


## FOREIGN STUDENTS

To be admitted to a recognized chiropractic college within the United States, students who are not U.S. citizens must:

1. Have the endorsement of the chiropractic organization of her or his home country if such an organization exists.

2. Submit proof of proficiency in the English language. A common method of establishing proficiency in English is through testing by the Institution for International Education or the U.S. State Department.

3. Submit evidence of having the financial resources, or funding commitment, to complete a minimum of one year of education.

4. Meet the same educational requirements as a student matriculating from the United States.

5. Have the transcript evaluated by a CCE-designated agency. An official copy of the evaluation will be forwarded directly to the institution and the student.

## HANDICAPPED STUDENTS

Handicapped students are treated no differently than other students. They are not denied admission because of their handicap, nor are there any special scholastic requirements. On the other hand, special scholastic or other types of privileges are rarely provided. For example, visually handicapped students will be required to carry out laboratory assignments, including microscopic work and roentgenographic interpretation. If this cannot be accomplished or if they cannot pass oral, written, and practical examinations and meet all of the requirements of the college, they cannot graduate. Thus, if unsurmountable problems can be anticipated, enrollment is not recommended.

## STUDENT ORIENTATION

During the first week of the opening semester, most all colleges conduct orientation sessions for first-year students as a means of conditioning new students to their new environment. These orientation sessions typically include discussions of the institution's objectives, organizational structure, procedures, scholastic regulations, student demeanor, student complaint procedures, requirements for successful completion of class work, class promotion, and graduation requirements.

Emphasis is usually given to defining a student's position in relation to the profession, including an explanation of the legal, economic, and social place of the profession within society. In addition, students are given an understanding of state regulations of the profession and the role of the examining boards, both as a protection of the public and the practitioners licensed to practice.

## CURRICULUM

The purpose of the curriculum is to provide the means for giving a student a thorough understanding of the structure and function of the human organism in health and disease. A well-balanced presentation is given the student so that he or she will have an understanding of the essential features of life processes in health and disease. Digestion, metabolism, excretion, physical and mental growth, nutrition, energy, nervous control, the significance of development defects, human behavior, and other elements are fundamental to the understanding of pathologic conditions. An understanding of structure and function makes it possible for students to identify deviations from the normal and provides the essential facts required in practice for diagnosis, treatment, or referral.

*Length, Sequence, and Depth of Course.* The curriculum in a recognized chiropractic college is presented over a minimum period of eight semesters or the equivalent for a total of not less than 4,200 hours. This comprehensive course of instruction is presented in a proper sequence of subjects to insure necessary prerequisites. The courses offered are taught in sufficient depth to fulfill the concept of the chiropractic physician as set forth in educational standards.

*Subjects.* Offerings within the curriculum typically include the following disciplines:

Anatomy (gross and histologic)
Biochemistry
Bioinstrumentation
Biomechanics and kinesiology
Clinical diagnosis
Clinical philosophy
Dermatology
Dietetics
Embryology
Emergency care
Endocrinology
Ethics and jurisprudence
Genetics
Gynecology
Histopathology
Laboratory diagnosis
Microbiology
Neurology
Nutrition
Office management and economics
Orthopedics
Otolaryngology
Pathology
Pediatrics
Physical diagnosis
Physiologic therapeutics
Physiology
Principles and practice of chiropractic
Psychology
Psychotherapeutics
Public health
Research methodology
Roentgenology and roentgenography
Symptomatology
Toxicology
Other appropriate subjects

## ACADEMIC STANDING AND GRADING

In the typical chiropractic college, a grade of 70 is considered passing in a course, but a cumulative average of 75 (2.0 GPA) for the semester must be maintained to remain in good standing.

Every effort is made by the various instructors to assist students who are experiencing difficulty with the work. If it is determined that the student does not possess the aptitude and is unable to make satisfactory progress or is unwilling to cooperate with offered faculty assistance, the student will be advised to withdraw from the college.

## GRADING SYSTEM

| Grade | Range | Grade Point (per semester hour) |
|-------|-------|--------------------------------|
| A | 95–100 | 4.0 |
| B+ | 90–94 | 3.5 |
| B | 85–89 | 3.0 |
| C+ | 80–84 | 2.5 |
| C | 75–79 | 2.0 |
| D | 70–74 | 1.0 |
| F | Below 70 | 0.0 |
| Incomplete | | |

## PROBATION AND SUSPENSION

Should a student's grade-point average fall below 2.0, or should there be as many as two failures during any one semester, the student is placed on academic probation in the typical chiropractic college. To be removed from probation, the student must earn a minimum grade-point average of 2.0 for the next semester and must demonstrate a cumulative grade-point average of 2.0.

A student beginning a semester on probation and failing to attain a 2.0 for that semester is usually subject to suspension. Should a student earn a grade-point average below 1.0 for a semester, or fail three courses in a semester, the student is subject to suspension.

Students readmitted after suspension continue on probation and may be denied advanced standing until all deficiencies are satisfactorily corrected, unless given permission by the academic dean. A student is rarely readmitted after a second suspension.

## EXAMINATIONS

All students are expected to take all examinations during a term. If an examination is missed for sufficient reason, a make-up examination may be given at the discretion of the instructor. For the second such make-up examination, a fee is usually required. Every effort should be made by the student to reach a mutually satisfactory arrangement with the instructor to take the examination within a period of two weeks following the date of the originally scheduled examination. In most instances, students will not be given the opportunity to make up more than two examinations in any one subject. Failure of an examination does not necessarily entitle a student to repeat the exam.

Final examinations are to be taken at the scheduled time unless special arrangements are made in advance with the instructor. Failure to take a final examination at the scheduled time usually subjects the student to a fee for any special final examinations administered.

## FAILURE OF SUBJECTS

Failure of a subject requires that the course be repeated. If the failure occurred due to failure of the final examination, a special repeat examination may be given with the approval of the instructor and the academic dean. The maximum possible grade on such an examination is usually 75. A charge is often required for this service.

## INCOMPLETES

A conditional grade of incomplete is usually given in a subject if the general average has been satisfactory but, for sufficient reason, a requirement of the course has not been met. The incomplete grade must be completed no later than two weeks into the next semester in most colleges. If not completed on time, the grade becomes a failure.

A student is not usually eligible to take the final examination in a subject for which he or she has not completed work. A charge may be required for special examination.

## CLASS ATTENDANCE

Regular and punctual attendance at all scheduled classes is expected of all students. A student my be dropped from a course or may receive a reduced grade for excessive absences. Three incidences of tardiness in most chiropractic colleges may, at the discretion of the instructor, constitute an absence.

## PROFESSIONAL ATTITUDE AND ATTIRE

Students are expected to present themselves as student doctors of chiropractic, both in attitude and appearance. The educational process at a chiropractic college is designed not only to teach the technical skills necessary for successful practice, but also to develop the professional image and attitude of a health care provider. To this end, students are expected to comply with standards of dress and appearance established by the college.

## DISCIPLINE

When a student is dropped from the rolls for absences, failing grades, or for misconduct, he or she may apply for readmission at the beginning of the next semester. The administration reserves the right to dismiss any student at the request of the faculty, the ethics committee, or at its own discretion. There is usually no refund of tuition in the case of such a dismissal.

## STUDENT GUIDANCE AND COUNSELING

The deans and faculty members in the chiropractic colleges make every effort to assist students with their problems and needs. Students are assigned to a faculty counselor and are encouraged to seek her or his assistance and guidance as necessary. In addition, administrative officers and consultants are available to help students with specific problems.

## COLLEGE LIBRARIES

Chiropractic college libraries provide a useful program of learning resource services for students, faculty, research personnel, and the profession in general. The resources and acquisitions exist for the purpose of training health care professionals and for developing a multimedia approach to augment and support the educational objectives.

Thousands of scientific volumes and hundreds of scientific and professional journals are available to enhance the educational and research objectives of the college. Audio-visual aids and equipment for student and staff use are available in all the basic and clinical sciences.

## COLLEGE LABORATORIES

In the typical chiropractic college, laboratories are designed for teaching, research, and patient diagnosis. Laboratory instruction is provided in gross anatomy, biomechanics, physiology, pathology, microbiology, chemistry, chiropractic technique, histology, clinical laboratory diagnosis, electrocardiography, physical diagnosis, physical therapy, and roentgenology. In addition, the college usually has one or more research laboratories for continuing research.

## COLLEGE CLINICS

Each college has one or more outpatient clinics for training junior and senior interns. The facilities are equipped with a variety of standard and research-oriented analytic, diagnostic, and therapeutic equipment designed to offer modern health care services. Lounges are usually available for both interns and staff doctors.

## STUDENT BENEFITS

Chiropractic health services are provided for all students in the outpatient clinic(s). Special rates are available for the families of married students.

As a member of the student ACA, the student is eligible to participate in professional group insurance at nominal fees.

## STUDENT ACA

This organization is affiliated with the American Chiropractic Association. It gives each member a four-year start in becoming a part of the profession. It attempts to give each member a greater understanding of what is occurring in the profession on local, state, and national levels.

Incorporated in this organization are representatives of each class, who act as members of a governing committee and council for student government. Membership dues in the student ACA are nominal. The student receives the *ACA Journal of Chiropractic* each month and other ACA publications.

## STUDENT ORGANIZATIONS

College administrations feel that student participation in organizational and group activities is of value in developing professional responsibility and attitudes. Through these activities, students become conditioned to their obligations to the profession to support its colleges and its local, state, and national organizations for professional growth.

## COLLEGE FRATERNITIES AND SORORITIES

These social organizations are engaged in promoting good fellowship, social recreation, and professional responsibilities. They are frequently involved in charitable projects within the community, developing special educational programs and assisting the college to meet special goals. Membership is by invitation.

## COLLEGE HONORARY SOCIETY

Membership in the college honorary society is open to those who maintain an academic standard of 3.5 or above for two consecutive semesters. Its purpose is to honor those students who have attained a high level of scholastic achievement. The obligations of its members are to exemplify the chiropractic image and aid those who need scholastic assistance.

## COLLEGE ATHLETIC CLUB

The typical chiropractic college has an athletic club, with faculty counseling and support, that arranges for participation in area-sponsored basketball, softball, and other athletic programs. Participation, based on sufficient student interest, is available in a variety of competitive activities including bowling, golf, tennis, volleyball, soccer, horseshoes, and table tennis. Recreational facilities for a number of sports and recreational activities are usually available on campus.

The more the chiropractic student actively participates in athletic events, the more he or she will be able to appreciate human biomechanics and the causes and implications of athletic and recreational injuries. Students soon realize that amateur athletes and weekend recreation enthusiasts do not protect themselves against spinal problems as do professionals. Proper health counsel is best given when founded upon personal experience.

## INSTITUTIONAL RECOGNITIONS

Chiropractic colleges are recognized throughout the nation at both the federal and state levels.

On the federal level, the U.S. Department of Education recognizes those colleges having status with the CCE and so lists them in its education directory. Certified chiropractic colleges are eligible for guaranteed student loans, NDSL, student work-study programs, and interest assistance programs. Chiropractic is listed in the *Occupational Outlook Handbook* of the U.S. Department of Labor. Chiropractic colleges are eligible for loans from the U.S. Department of Housing and Urban Development. In addition, the Veterans Administration recognizes chiropractic institutions as institutions of higher education, and student visas for chiropractic students are granted by the U.S. Department of Immigration and Naturalization.

On the national level, a substantial number of accredited colleges in various states include a prechiropractic curriculum in their catalogs, and it is not uncommon to transfer credit from chiropractic colleges to regionally accredited institutions. Several chiropractic colleges have established cooperative programs with regionally accredited institutions of higher education.

## PROFESSIONAL WORKFORCE NEEDS

Trends show the need for greater numbers of doctors of chiropractic. Opportunities for chiropractic physicians are expected to be very good through the next few decades. Some communities are without any D.C. practitioners, and many more have an inadequate number. In addition, many more new practitioners will be necessary to replace those who retire or die.

The chiropractic profession is expected to grow faster than the average for all occupations through the 1980s because of population growth, an increasing number of persons receiving chiropractic services, an increasing number of patient visits, and the expansion of prepaid health care programs such as Medicare, Medicaid, state, and private health plans.

A 1978 Missouri Manpower Study determined that the "adequate and acceptable" workforce level for the state was twenty-five active practitioners per 100,000 persons. Projected to the national level, this would suggest a need of about 55,000 practitioners. At the present time, there are about 30,000 active practitioners in the United States.

## CONTINUING EDUCATION

Recognizing that any healing art must keep abreast of new data and procedures, the chiropractic profession has supported continuing education as a yearly requirement for licensure in forty-one jurisdictions. More states are supporting this effort each year.

Voluntary programs are another important part of chiropractic continuing education. Each accredited chiropractic college maintains an ongoing postgraduate (continuing) education division whose objective is to provide postgraduate education to better assist the doctor of chiropractic in the care of the public. Each postgraduate division or department produces programs, courses, and seminars that are designed to upgrade the competence, knowledge, and ability of graduate doctors of chiropractic.

The ACA Council on Athletics and Physical Fitness, Council on Orthopedics, Council on Roentgenology, and

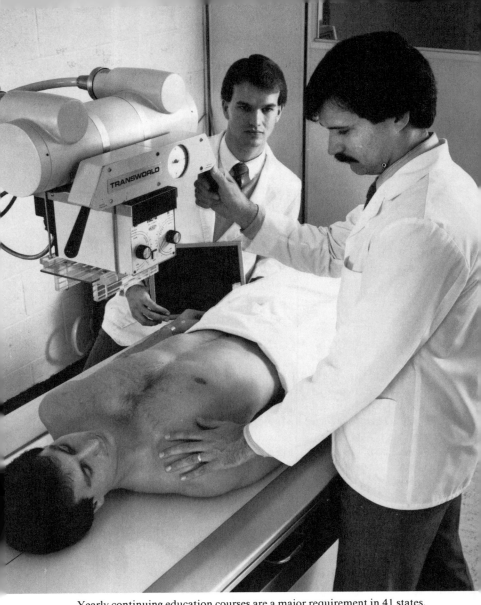

Yearly continuing education courses are a major requirement in 41 states. Courses covering advances in X-ray diagnosis and other skills lead to specialized certification and/or diplomate status.

Council on Nutrition have programs leading to certification and/or diplomate status. Other ACA councils offer postgraduate educational programs to enhance the practitioner's continuing education.

In addition, state chiropractic associations periodically offer educational programs for the benefit of their members. These programs are frequently supplemented at the local level by programs conducted by chiropractic researchers and clinicians.

## CONSIDERATIONS INVOLVED IN ESTABLISHING A PRACTICE

After students have been graduated from a chiropractic college as a doctor of chiropractic, passed the required state board examinations, and received a license, they are now ready to set up practice. The new doctor will be confronted by several alternatives: (1) to set up a new office, (2) purchase an established practice, or (3) join an established practitioner or group practice.

The new doctor will need to obtain equipment which he or she will have learned to use while earning the D.C. degree. Every chiropractic office needs chairs and tables for the reception room. This equipment often comes with the office. Equipment such as an X-ray machine, other diagnostic equipment, treatment tables, and similar items can cost from $30,000 to $50,000. Because of this enormous expense, there are firms who will arrange with the new chiropractic to purchase all the equipment and then lease it or let the doctor pay in installments over several years.

A chiropractic can incorporate her or his practice, although fewer than one in ten do so. This gives the doctor certain legal and tax advantages in some cases.

The new doctor can also purchase an established practice. For example, announcements in chiropractic journals frequently offer a fully established practice for sale, including a furnished office and equipment. This option has advantages and disadvantages. The advantages are that the new doctor can begin practice in possession of most of the essential equipment. On the other hand, the new doctor may find the retiring physician's equipment outdated. In addition, there is no assurance that the new doctor will inherit all the patients of the retiring doctor.

The new doctor may decide to go into practice with an already established physician, using the same office and equipment and seeing some of the established doctor's patients. Or the new doctor may decide to make an arrangement that will permit use of another professional's office during hours when that doctor isn't there.

There are many alternatives to starting a practice, but that is often the only alternative for many chiropractors. In some remote areas of the country, there isn't an established practice for a new doctor to take over even if he or she so wished. Because of the severe shortage of chiropractic physicians, many of them are located in cities. If a new doctor wants a country or small town practice, it will sometimes be necessary to set it up from scratch.

When a new doctor enters a partnership, he or she agrees to share expenses and income with another chiropractic physician. Obviously, this arrangement only works well in a community large enough to provide a sufficient number of patients for both doctors.

Sometimes a new doctor may decide to join a chiropractic group practice. This arrangement is a popular one because practitioners of the chiropractic art can group together in one building with adequate parking and share a receptionist, some of the equipment and facilities, as well as the chiropractic paraprofessionals on the staff. Overhead costs can be greatly reduced in this manner.

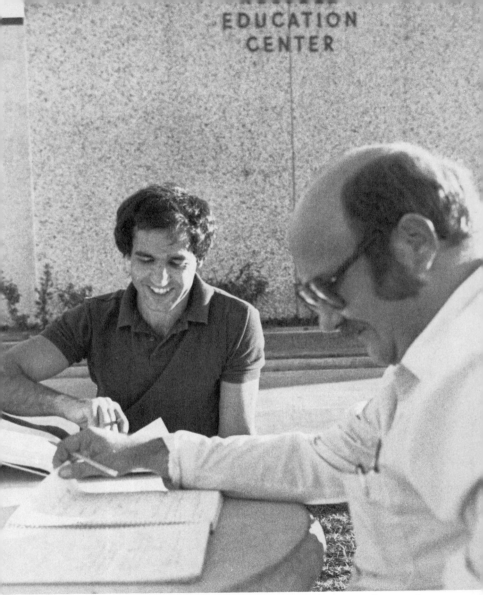

Because chiropractic health care is being included in more and more private and public health care programs, the chiropractic professional can expect a bright future of growth and expansion in this field.

# CHAPTER 6

# THE FUTURE OF CHIROPRACTIC

For those seeking a career in the chiropractic profession, the future looks very bright. Several years ago, Orval L. Hidde, D.C., J.D., suggested that, in the future, chiropractic physicians may be on the staffs of hospitals and other public institutions, included in all public health policy-making decisions, and the recipients of additional funds for research. Many of these predictions have already become realities.

Each year, chiropractic services are being included in more and more state and federal health programs. Doctors of chiropractic are actively cooperating with state health planning commissions in the development of health programs and services. Cost-effectiveness studies showing chiropractic benefits have done much to establish recognition of chiropractic as an efficient form of health care.

With the push toward higher educational standards, the Foundation for Chiropractic Education and Research has made over $300,000 a year available for awards and grants. Research facilities are also being upgraded and expanded in all chiropractic colleges recognized by the CCE.

## OPPORTUNITIES FOR MINORITIES

Although only a small percentage of blacks, Hispanics, American Indians, and other minority groups have entered chiropractic, they are welcomed by the profession. The reason for today's small representation of minorities is probably due to a lack of effort on the part of high schools to interest such students in this special area. Another reason is that in past years, public school conditions were not always conducive to offering quality science courses to sufficiently prepare students for the study of medicine. Fortunately, today the trend is to develop community colleges throughout the country which offer strong remedial programs to assist minority groups with compensatory education to help bridge this gap. Counselors on all levels now point out the desirability of a chiropractic career to interested members of minority groups.

Although a student may gain admission to many chiropractic colleges with a minimum of two years of college preparation (which could be obtained in many good community colleges), the student might do better with even more advanced educational preparation, such as three or four years. In fact, about 40 percent of the students now entering chiropractic college have a bachelor's degree. Many practitioners believe that in the near future a bachelor's degree will be the minimum requirement for entrance into an accredited college of chiropractic.

## RECOGNITION BY FEDERAL, STATE, AND PRIVATE AGENCIES

All fifty states, plus the District of Columbia, Puerto Rico, and several foreign countries, license and officially recognize chiropractic as a health profession. All fifty states authorize chiropractic services as part of their worker's compensation program.

By congressional action and with presidential approval, chiropractic is authorized and recognized for all Americans in Medicare, Medicaid, and the Vocational Rehabilitation Program. Under the Internal Revenue Code, chiropractic care is a medical deduction. Specifically for federal employees, chiropractic is included in 13 of the 17 organization plans in the Federal Employee health programs. The Railroad Retirement Act, the Longshoremen's and Harbor Worker's Compensation Act as well as the Federal Employees Compensation Act include chiropractic services.

The U.S. Public Health Service classifies doctors of chiropractic among "medical specialists and practitioners," includes D.C.s in its *Health Manpower Sourcebook,* and includes a chapter covering chiropractic in *Health Resources Statistics.* The U.S. Department of Labor lists chiropractic in its *Occupational Outlook Handbook.*

In the private sector, virtually all major health insurance carriers include chiropractic in their private policies. About 65 percent of the states require inclusion of chiropractic services under all commercial health and accident policies written in those states. Also, the National Conference of Insurance Legislators adopted a model bill for state health insurance programs that defines "physician" to include doctor of chiropractic.

Major industrial employers such as General Motors have included chiropractic in their health plan for employees. In addition, a substantial number of major international, national, and local unions include chiropractic in their health and welfare plans.

## COST-EFFECTIVENESS STUDIES

Studies of worker's compensation records provide objective evidence of the efficacy of chiropractic health care in the treatment of industrial injuries. From data supplied by Workmen's Compensation Commissions, comparisons of D.C. and M.D. treatment of industrial injuries have demonstrated dramatically that those cases under chiropractic care showed (1) reduced treatment costs, (2) reduced compensation costs, (3) reduced work-time losses, and (4) reduced disability and suffering.

*Florida.* A Florida study indicates that treatment costs for substantially identical cases were 27.5 percent less for cases handled by D.C.s than for cases handled by M.D.s. The study also found that when back and neck injuries were treated by medical doctors, as compared to similar injuries treated by doctors of chiropractic, (a) compensation costs averaged 211 percent more ($37 vs. $9), and (b) work-time losses averaged 200 percent more (9 days vs. 3 days).

*Oregon.* The medical director of the Workmen's Compensation Board of the State of Oregon released the results of a similar study, "A Study of Time Loss Back Claims, 1977," which showed that of claimants treated by no other physician than a chiropractor, 82 percent of those workers resumed work after one week of time loss. These claims were closed without a disability award. However, among claimants treated by M.D. s, in which the diagnosis seems comparable to the type of injury suffered by the workers treated by the D.C., only 41 percent of these workers resumed work after one week of time loss.

In a separate study of statistical information furnished by the Oregon Workmen's Compensation Board in 1971, a twenty-four-month study limited to back-injury cases involving sprains and strains only found: $298.52 average total cost under care of M.D.s, as compared to only $72.92 average total cost under care of D.C.s. These average total costs include doctor and hospital costs plus compensable time loss.

*Kansas.* A comparative study of Kansas worker's compensation records in 1972 of average time loss and treatment costs for back injuries handled by doctors of chiropractic and medical doctors is shown in Table 2.

**TABLE 2. AVERAGE TIME LOSS AND TREATMENT COSTS**
(Kansas 1972)

|  | Time Lost | Treatment Costs (excluding hospital costs) |
|---|---|---|
| M.D. Care ... | 11.4 days per case | $103.10 per case |
| D.C. Care ... | 5.8 days per case | $ 68.43 per case |

*Iowa.* A comparison of the cost of D.C. vs. M.D. treatment is found in two Iowa studies covering the years 1966 and 1969. Average cost per case for M.D. treatment in 1966 was $118.74 and $210.86 in 1969, as compared to average cost per case for D.C. care of $68.24 in 1966 and $79.28 in 1969.

An analysis in 1978 of nonoperative back and neck injury claims processed by the Office of the Industrial Commissioner reported that both the average period of disability and the average amount of compensation awarded were lower for chiropractic patients than for medical patients. Appearing in Table 3 is a comparison of average length of disability and average compensation cost per case experienced by claimants of various groups in that study.

**TABLE 3. AVERAGE PERIOD OF DISABILITY
AND COMPENSATION PAID**
(Iowa 1978)

| Age Group | Chiropractic | | Medical | |
|---|---|---|---|---|
| | Disability (days) | Compensation Paid | Disability (days) | Compensation Paid |
| 16–24 yrs | 21.1 | $204.16 | 25.3 | $319.20 |
| 25–44 yrs | 22.4 | 284.79 | 24.4 | 353.62 |
| Over 44 yrs | 21.7 | 258.61 | 27.1 | 423.34 |
| All Ages | 21.9 | $262.21 | 25.1 | $360.06 |

*California.* In December 1972, C. Richard Wolf, M.D., completed a study which was designed to compare time loss due to industrial back injury when treated by either a D.C. or an M.D., using the records of the Division of Labor Statistics and Research (Doctor's First Report of Work Injury). In summary, 1000 employees with industrial back injuries were questioned about the time lost and residual pain suffered from injuries. One-half of this group had been treated by M.D. and one-half by D.C. physicians. Of the 1000 employees surveyed, 629 responded to the questionnaire. No degree of bias in study design could be determined, and there were no apparent major identifiable differences in the two groups with regard to age or employee categories. The major differences determined are shown in Table 4.

**TABLE 4. AVERAGE TIME LOST AND RECOVERY**
(California 1972)

|  | Employees Treated by M.D.s | Employees Treated by D.C.s |
|---|---|---|
| Average lost time per employee ....... | 32 days | 15.6 days |
| Employees reporting no lost time .... | 21.0% | 47.9% |
| Employees reporting lost time in excess of 60 days ..................... | 13.2% | 6.7% |
| Employees reporting complete recovery ........................................ | 34.8% | 51.0% |

*Montana.* In 1978, a comparison on chiropractic and medical ambulatory care of back strain and sprain injuries in Montana from 1975 to 1978 was made. The average period of disability and average amount of compensation paid to chiropractic and medical patients with back strain and sprain injuries are shown in Table 5.

**TABLE 5. COMPARATIVE D.C. AND M.D. DATA**
(Montana 1978)

| Age Group | D.C. Patients Disability (weeks) | Compensation Paid | M.D./D.O. Patients Disability (weeks) | Compensation Paid |
|---|---|---|---|---|
| 16–24 yrs | 3.0 | $378.35 | 3.3 | $466.71 |
| 25–44 yrs | 1.8 | 248.60 | 3.0 | 409.83 |
| Over 44 yrs | 3.8 | 352.98 | 5.9 | 561.04 |
| All Ages | 2.8 | $315.93 | 4.0 | $463.66 |

*Wisconsin.* Also in 1978, Daniel J. Duffy, M.B.A., in Market Research, University of Wisconsin, conducted a comparative study of M.D. vs. D.C. treatment of closed industrial back injury cases for 1977. The results are shown in Table 6.

**TABLE 6. COMPARATIVE D.C. AND M.D. DATA**
(Wisconsin 1978)

|  | Cases | Days Lost | Treatment Costs |
|---|---|---|---|
| M.D. Care ...... | 430 | 21.8 | $267.58 |
| D.C. Care ....... | 212 | 13.2 | 145.64 |

## THE FOUNDATION FOR CHIROPRACTIC EDUCATION AND RESEARCH (FCER)

The Foundation for Chiropractic Education and Research (FCER) is a nonprofit organization established by the profession in 1944 to further the growth and development of the chiropractic profession. As the profession's primary source of financial support for chiropractic research, FCER seeks to ensure chiropractic's acceptance as a major science-based health-care profession.

In addition to receiving an annual grant from the American Chiropractic Association, FCER's programs are supported by thousands of active members including doctors, patients, suppliers, state associations and their auxiliaries, and other individuals. Contributions made in the form of general contributions, membership dues, memorials, bequests through wills, and major planned gifts are applied to the Foundation's many research programs.

Since establishing its Awards and Grants Program in 1980,

FCER has supported approximately 70 key research projects at 13 chiropractic colleges and many other academic and research institutions around the world.

Findings resulting from these studies have been published in respected scientific and professional journals, and numerous presentations have been made at major conferences both within and outside of the chiropractic profession.

FCER's Awards and Grants Program supports basic and clinical research at chiropractic colleges and major universities throughout the world. This program also funds fellowships for the training of chiropractic doctors pursuing advanced degrees in scientific and nonclinical health-related areas, and it provides grants-in-aid of dissertation research for students enrolled in doctoral programs in clinical biomechanics.

Grant applications received by the Foundation are rigorously judged on their scientific merit and relevance to chiropractic against standards and procedures consistent with other well-established funding organizations and federal agencies.

Over the past several years, FCER-supported research has included the following areas: evaluation of the effects of chiropractic spinal manipulation as a treatment for a variety of neuromusculoskeletal and other health disorders; analysis of the biomechanical aspects of the human spine; determination of the accuracy and usefulness of radiographic assessments of vertebral alignment; quantification of occupational and demographic factors that lead to low-back pain; and examination of the utilization patterns of chiropractic health care services.

## 1986: A NEW DIRECTION

To maintain its leadership role in the developing health-care field, FCER embarked on an ambitious new research program in 1986.

This new program emphasizes observable and measurable scientific outcomes that are of great importance to the chiropractic profession. Specifically, this program focuses on the profession's three most commonly treated health problems—low back pain, headaches, and sports-related injuries. At the core of this new program are large-scale clinical studies.

## EDUCATION AND TRAINING

FCER assigns a high priority to fellowship awards for the post-doctoral training of chiropractors. Numerous awards have been made to chiropractors enrolled in master's or doctoral programs. Their areas of study have included biomechanics, anatomy, physiology, public health, and epidemiology. Many FCER Fellows have gone on to make significant contributions to the scientific research literature in chiropractic.

Because the involvement of the chiropractic colleges is critical to chiropractic research, FCER maintains close ties with these colleges. The assistance the Foundation has given the chiropractic colleges through research grants has enabled them to strengthen and, in some instances, establish significant research programs.

## THE CHIROPRACTIC RESEARCH COMMISSION

In 1977, FCER established the Chiropractic Research Commission (CRC). Comprised of the research directors of the chiropractic colleges, the CRC meets to discuss common concerns and issues. These meetings give college leaders the opportunity to discuss education and research goals, and identify and find solutions to problems they experience.

In 1982, the CRC organized the profession's first scientific research conference. Now held annually, the Conservative Health Science Research Conferences are the primary means by which chiropractic researchers report their findings to the scientific community.

FCER also established a Student Research Awards Program in 1986 to recognize chiropractic students who demonstrate a strong personal commitment to research. Based on papers submitted to FCER, three students are selected annually for awards.

## THE FEDERATION OF CHIROPRACTIC LICENSING BOARDS (FCLB)

The FCLB is composed of representatives from the various state boards concerned with the examination and licensing of chiropractic applicants. It is affiliated with the Federation of Associations of Health Regulatory Boards. Each year, the FCLB publishes an updated *Official Directory of Chiropractic & Basic Science Examining Boards with Licensure & Practice Statistics.*

Questions relative to basic statistical information should be directed to: Cynthia E. Preiss, D.C., F.I.C.C., Secretary-Treasurer, FCLB, 501 East California Avenue, Glendale, California 91206.

## THE AMERICAN CHIROPRACTIC ASSOCIATION (ACA)

The ACA is a national nonprofit professional membership organization, which has a working relationship with state chiropractic associations. Its major income comes from dues and publication sales. The ACA conducts the customary professional activities of a national health professional association.

As of 1986–87, the ACA had over 23,000 members, representing the vast majority of licensed practitioners in the United States. The ACA serves as national spokesman for the profession. A primary objective of the organization is to establish and maintain the ethics and professional competency necessary or desirable to meet the requirements of the profession and the expectations of society.

1. *Councils.* There are ACA-sponsored professional councils for diagnosis and internal disorders, mental health, neurology, nutrition, orthopedics, physiotherapy, roentgenology, and sports injuries.
2. *Related Agencies.* Related agencies include such organizations as the American Chiropractic Auxiliary and Foundation for Chiropractic Education and Research.
3. *Technical Assistance.* Upon request, ACA provides counsel to practitioners working within the chiropractic profession and with other professions, and to government, health, industrial, insurance, and other groups with health-related interests.
4. *Educational Services.* The Association develops, produces, and distributes extensive materials on a wide variety of health subjects by such means as films, slide programs with taped narrations, pamphlets, booklets, texts, posters, displays, and kits. The *ACA Educational*

*Communications* price list indicates materials and supplies available as well as prices and ordering instructions. Also, vocational guidance materials are available. Periodically the ACA sponsors regional seminars and workshops designed to maintain the professional competency of practitioners, to coordinate research activities, and to introduce technological and scientific findings.

5. *Research.* The ACA contributes a substantial portion of its dues receipts to education and research through the facilities of the Foundation for Chiropractic Education and Research.

6. *Committees/Commissions.* The ACA maintains activities in such areas as senior citizens, student ACA, veteran affairs, health systems delivery, technic and procedures evaluation, labor relations, legislation, publications, public health, and radiological health.

7. *Major Health Education Activities.* By way of various communications media, the ACA seeks to provide information of value to public health, safety, physical fitness, and disease prevention. The following are examples of such programs:

(a) Radio and television public service announcements designed to increase public awareness of health concerns. Subjects include accident prevention, problems of the senior citizen, need for periodic health examinations, importance of correct posture and physical fitness, and other topics deemed important to national health.

(b) Public service billboards, newspaper health columns, space announcements, and news releases designed to call public attention to health matters of national concern.

(c) ACA Councils participate in workshops and continuing education in such areas as diagnosis and internal disorders, mental health, neurology, nutrition, orthopedics, physiotherapy, roentgenology, sports injuries, and chiropractic techniques.

(d) ACA supports the activities of the Foundation for Chiropractic Education and Research and the Council on Chiropractic Education.

(e) ACA sponsors "Correct Posture Month" in May of each year and "Spinal Health Month" in October of each year as continuing programs in health education.

(f) The Association serves as a national resource for current data and state of the art information relative to the profession and its contribution to public health.

## PROFESSIONAL COUNCILS, COMMISSIONS, AND COMMITTEES

Councils are formed to contribute to the efficient operation of the organization and are dedicated to a special area of interest in the field of chiropractic. Each council is composed of members in a specific field of chiropractic interested in working with others in the same specialized area through exchange of ideas, professional or technical papers, and general information.

The currently authorized councils are: (1) Council of Delegates, which is composed of elected state delegates and alternates in the ACA; (2) Council on Technic; (3) Council on Roentgenology; (4) Council on Mental Health; (5) Council on Orthopedics; (6) Council on Physiological Therapeutics; (7) Council on Neurology; (8) Council on Diagnosis and Internal Disorders; (9) Council on Sports Injuries and Physical Fitness; and (10) Council on Nutrition.

Within the ACA, various committees and commissions are authorized to perform specific duties by action of the house of delegates, the president, or the executive board of governors. The executive board of governors establishes the rules and regulations for the operation of all ACA committees and commissions, which may be revised as needed. These rules, objectives, and suggested action programs are subject to the approval of the house of delegates. Thus, democratic principles are upheld throughout the organizational structure.

In addition to several executive board committees, currently authorized general committees are the Advertising & Exhibits Committee, Awards Committee, Code of Ethics Committee, Committee on Senior Citizens, Student ACA Committee, Veteran Affairs Committee, Bylaws Committee, and the Resolutions Committee.

Five commissions are currently authorized by the ACA. These are the Commission on Health Delivery Systems, Commission on Industrial Relations, Commission on Insurance, Commission on Labor Relations, and Commission on Legislation.

As the names and addresses of council, committee, and commission officers are subject to change, requests for further information should be addressed to the specific group at the ACA's executive headquarters, 1701 Clarendon Boulevard, Arlington, Virginia 22209.

# STATE BOARDS OF CHIROPRACTIC EXAMINERS

*Alabama State Board of Chiropractic Examiners*
    P.O. Drawer 3607
    Robertsdale, AL 36567

*Alaska Board of Chiropractic Examiners*
    Department of Commerce
    Division of Occupational Licensing, Pouch D
    Juneau, AK 99811

*Arizona State Board of Chiropractic Examiners*
    Arizona Board of Chiropractic Examiners
    1645 West Jefferson, Room 471
    Phoenix, AZ 85007

*Arkansas State Board of Chiropractic Examiners*
    404 Southwest Avenue
    El Dorado, AR 71730

*California State Board of Chiropractic Examiners*
    921 11th Street, Suite 601
    Sacramento, CA 95814

*Colorado State Board of Chiropractic Examiners*
   1525 Sherman, Room 128
   State Services Building
   Denver, CO 80203

*Connecticut Board of Chiropractic Examiners*
   3466 Main Street
   Stratford, CT 06497

*Delaware State Board of Chiropractic Examiners*
   Office of Professional Licensing
   Margaret O'Neill Building
   Dover, DE 19901

*Board of Examiners in Chiropractic*
   605 G Street, Room 202, NW, Lower Level
   Washington, D.C. 20001

*Florida State Board of Chiropractic*
   Department of Professional Regulation
   130 N. Monroe Street
   Tallahassee, FL 32301

*Georgia Board of Chiropractic Examiners*
   State Examining Boards
   166 Pryor Street, S.W.
   Atlanta, GA 30303

*Hawaii Board of Chiropractic Examiners*
   Department of Commerce and Consumer Affairs
   P.O. Box 3469
   Honolulu, HI 96801

*Idaho State Board of Chiropractic Examiners*
   Rt. 1, Box 102C
   St. Maries, ID 83861

*Illinois Medical Examining Committee*
   6012 West Fullerton
   Chicago, IL 60639

*Indiana Board of Chiropractic Examiners*
Health Professions Service Bureau
700 N. High School Road
Indianapolis, IN 46224

*Iowa Board of Chiropractic Examiners*
State Department of Health
Lucas State Office Building
Des Moines, IA 50306

*Kansas State Board of Healing Arts*
503 Kansas Avenue, Suite 500
Topeka, KS 66603

*Kentucky State Board of Chiropractic Examiners*
209 East Main Street
Glasgow, KY 42141

*Louisiana Board of Chiropractic Examiners*
5501 Gardner Highway
Alexandria, LA 71301

*Maine Board of Chiropractic Examination & Registration*
51 Main Street
Springvale, ME 04083

*Maryland State Board of Chiropractic Examiners*
8003 Flower Avenue
Takoma Park, MD 20912

*Massachusetts Board of Registration of Chiropractors*
Room 1514, Leverett Saltonstall Building
100 Cambridge Street
Boston, MA 02202

*Michigan Board of Chiropractic*
Department of Licensing & Regulations
905 Southland, Box 30018
Lansing, MI 48909

*Minnesota State Board of Chiropractic Examiners*
    717 Delaware Street, S.E., Room 336
    Minneapolis, MN 55414

*Mississippi Board of Chiropractic Examiners*
    91 Lakeview Drive
    Clinton, MS 39056

*Missouri State Board of Chiropractic Examiners*
    P.O. Box 672
    Jefferson City, MO 65102-0672

*Board of Chiropractors*
    1424 9th Avenue
    Helena, MT 59620-0407

*Nebraska Chiropractic Board of Examiners*
    Department of Health
    Bureau of Examining Boards
    P.O. Box 95007
    Lincoln, NE 68509

*Nevada State Board of Chiropractic Examiners*
    P.O. Box 20582
    Reno, NV 89515

*New Hampshire State Board of Chiropractic Examiners &
    Regulation*
    58 East Dunstable Road
    Nashua, NH 03060

*New Jersey State Board of Medical Examiners*
    940 Avenue "C"
    Bayonne, NJ 07002

*New Mexico State Board of Chiropractic Examiners*
    P.O. Box 1763
    Alamogordo, NM 88311-1763

*New York State Board for Chiropractic*
    State Education Department
    Cultural Education Center
    Albany, NY 12230

*North Carolina State Board of Chiropractic Examiners*
    P.O. Box 312
    Concord, NC 28025

*North Dakota Board of Chiropractic Examiners*
    1415 2nd Avenue, S.W.
    Minot, ND 58701

*Ohio State Board of Chiropractic Examiners*
    200 E. Town Street
    Columbus, OH 43215

*Oklahoma Board of Chiropractic Examiners*
    2401 S.W. 45th Street
    Oklahoma City, OK 73119

*Oregon State Board of Chiropractic Examiners*
    P.O. Box 20455
    Portland, OR 97220

*Pennsylvania State Board of Chiropractic Examiners*
    Department of State
    Bureau of Professional & Occupational Affairs
    P.O. Box 2649
    Harrisburg, PA 17105

*Puerto Rico Board of Chiropractic Examiners*
    McArthur Street, No. 10
    Old San Juan, PR 00901

*Rhode Island State Board of Chiropractic Examiners*
    Division of Professional Regulation
    104 Cannon Building
    Davis Street
    Providence, RI 02908

*South Carolina Board of Chiropractic Examiners*
   P.O. Box 711
   Kingstree, SC 29556

*South Dakota State Board of Chiropractic Examiners*
   Box 37
   Marion, SD 57043

*Tennessee State Board of Chiropractic Examiners*
   Tennessee Dept. of Public Health
   State Office Building
   Ben Allen Road
   Nashville, TN 37216

*Texas Board of Chiropractic Examiners*
   1300 E. Anderson Lane, Bldg. C, Suite 245
   Austin, TX 78752

*Utah State Chiropractors Examining Committee*
   Division of Registration
   Room 500
   State Office Building
   Salt Lake City, UT 84114

*Vermont State Board of Chiropractic Examination &*
   *Registration*
   45 Court Street
   Middlebury, VT 05753

*The Virginia Board of Medicine*
   1932 Arlington Blvd.
   Charlottesville, VA 22903

*Washington State Board of Chiropractic Examiners*
   3810 Steilacoom Blvd.
   Tacoma, WA 98499

*West Virginia Board of Chiropractic Examiners*
   142 McCorkle Avenue
   St. Albans, WV 25177

*Wisconsin Chiropractic Examining Board*
    2019 Main Street
    Whitehall, WI 54773

*Wyoming State Board of Chiropractic Examiners*
    Box 453
    Mt. View, WY 82939

## APPENDIX B

# CHIROPRACTIC ASSOCIATIONS

*American Chiropractic Association*
Executive Headquarters
1701 Clarendon Boulevard
Arlington, VA 22209

*Council on Chiropractic Education*
Executive Headquarters
3209 Ingersoll, Suite 206
Des Moines, IA 50312

*Federation of Chiropractic Licensing Boards*
501 East California Avenue
Glendale, CA 91206

*Foundation for Chiropractic Education and Research*
Executive Headquarters
1701 Clarendon Boulevard
Arlington, VA 22209

*National Board of Chiropractic Examiners*
Executive Headquarters
1610 29th Avenue Place
Greeley, CO 80631

## APPENDIX C

# TYPICAL CHIROPRACTIC CURRICULUM

## GENERAL INFORMATION

Chiropractic college courses are set up on either the trimester or quarterly basis. In either case, the four-year course can be completed in less than four calendar years if students choose to continue their education through the summer months. Both trimester and the quarterly systems provide for this option.

### Typical Trimester Calendar

The trimester course, utilized by the majority of colleges, is typically concluded in 10 trimesters of about 15 weeks each, which can be completed consecutively in 3.3 calendar years. Approximately a two-week recess is allowed between trimesters. A typical calendar would be:

Fall trimester . . . . . . . . . . . . Sep   1–Dec 15
Recess  . . . . . . . . . . . . . . . . Dec 16–Jan   1
Spring trimester . . . . . . . . . Jan   2–Apr 15
Recess  . . . . . . . . . . . . . . . . Apr 16–Apr 30

134

Summer trimester . . . . . . . .  May   1–Aug 15
Recess . . . . . . . . . . . . . . . .  Aug 16–Aug 31

## Typical Quarterly Calendar

The quarterly course is typically concluded in 12 quarters of about 12 weeks each, which can be completed consecutively in three calendar years. A short vacation period is allowed between the Spring and Summer quarters and a Christmas recess is provided between the Fall and Winter quarters. A typical calendar would be:

Winter quarter . . . . . . . . . . .  Jan   6–Mar 21
Spring quarter . . . . . . . . . . .  Mar 24–Jun  13
Summer recess . . . . . . . . . . .  Jun  14–Jly   13
Summer quarter . . . . . . . . .  Jly   14–Oct   3
Fall quarter . . . . . . . . . . . . .  Oct   6–Dec  19
Christmas recess . . . . . . . . .  Dec 20–Jan   5

## DEGREE CURRICULUM

### Typical Trimester Curriculum

*Trimester 1*

Spinal anatomy
Spinal anatomy lab
Osteology
Osteology lab
Myology
Myology lab
Terminology
Physiology I

Chiropractic principles I
Principles of biochemistry
Biochemistry lab
General microbiology
General microbiology lab
Neuroanatomy
Palpation I lab
First aid and minor surgery

*Trimester 2*

Regional anatomy
Dissection I lab

Circulation
Human biochemistry

Embryology
Physiology II
Physiology lab I
Endocrinology

Pathologic microbiology
Chiropractic principles II
Spinal biomechanics
Palpation II with lab

*Trimester 3*

Regional anatomy II
Dissection II lab
Histology
Histology lab
Physiology III
Physiology lab II
Human genetics

Public health
Emergency health care
  with lab
Chiropractic principles III
Adjusting procedures I
Adjusting procedures I lab

*Trimester 4*

General pathology
Pathology lab
Clinical neurology
Principles of diagnosis
Neurologic-orthopedic
  examination
Neurologic-orthopedic
  lab

Diagnosis I, physical
Principles/technique of X-ray
Principles/technique
  of X-ray lab
Research methodology
Adjusting procedures II
Adjusting procedures II lab

*Trimester 5*

Systems pathology
Diagnosis II, physical
Physical diagnosis lab
Clinical lab diagnosis
Dermatology
Cardiovascular disorders
Electrocardiology

Eye-ear-nose-throat disorders
Roentgenographic diagnosis I
Appendicular biomechanics
Clinical orientation
Toxicology
Adjusting procedures III
Adjusting procedures III lab

*Trimester 6*

Orthopedic diagnosis
Neurologic diagnosis
Pediatrics

Physical therapy I lab
Adjusting procedures IV
Adjusting procedures IV lab

Nutrition I

Obstetrics and gynecology

Professional ethics

Physical therapy I

Roentgenographic diagnosis II

Clinic I

*Trimester 7*

The digestive system

The respiratory system

The genitourinary system

Abnormal psychology

Nutrition II

Physical therapy II

Physical therapy II lab

Spinal orthopedics

Appendicular orthopedics

Appendicular orthopedics lab

Health care insurance

Adjusting procedures V

Adjusting procedures V lab

Clinic II

*Trimester 8*

Geriatrics

Roentgenographic diagnosis III

Appendicular orthopedics II

Appendicular orthopedics II lab

Jurisprudence

Case management I

Clinic management I

Adjusting procedures VI

Adjusting procedures VI lab

Clinic III

*Trimester 9*

Roentgenographic diagnosis IV

Office management

Case management II

Immunogenesis

Rehabilitation

Clinic management II

Adjusting procedures VII

Adjusting procedures VII lab

Traumatology

Clinic IV

*Trimester 10*

Preceptorship

Clinic V

## Typical Quarterly Curriculum

*Quarter 1—Freshman I*

| | |
|---|---|
| Myology | Histology |
| Myology lab | Histology lab |
| Osteology | Embryology |
| Osteology lab | Biophysics |
| Arthrology | Philosophy I |

*Quarter 2—Freshman II*

| | |
|---|---|
| Splanchnology | Biochemistry I |
| Angiology | Biomechanics |
| Cellular physiology | Palpation |
| Cellular physiology lab | Philosophy II |

*Quarter 3—Freshman III*

| | |
|---|---|
| Central neurology | Hematology lab |
| Biochemistry II | Roentgenology |
| Cardiovascular | Spinal anatomy |
| physiology | Adjusting procedures I |
| General pathology I | Adjusting procedures I lab |
| Hematology | |

*Quarter 4—Sophomore I*

| | |
|---|---|
| Peripheral neurology | General pathology II |
| Biochemistry lab | Roentgenography I |
| Endocrinology | Roentgenography I lab |
| Nutrition | Adjusting procedures II |
| Dietetics | Adjusting procedures II lab |

*Quarter 5—Sophomore II*

| | |
|---|---|
| Special senses | Public health |
| Neurophysiology | Adjusting procedures III |
| Physiologic chemistry | Adjusting procedures III lab |
| Toxicology | Elective |

*Quarter 6—Sophomore III*

| | |
|---|---|
| Dissection lab | Neuromusculoskeletal |
| Topography | pathology I |

Digestion physiology
Nutrition physiology
Renal physiology
Pulmonary physiology
Philosophy III

Roentgenography II
Roentgenography II lab
Adjusting procedures IV
Adjusting procedures IV lab

*Quarter 7—Junior I*

Physiology lab
Cardiovascular pathology
Gastrointestinal
pathology
Urogenital pathology
Neuromusculoskeletal
pathology II

Physics of roentgenology
Adjusting procedures V
Adjusting procedures V lab
Roentgenography III
Roentgenography III lab

*Quarter 8—Junior II*

Physical diagnosis
Roentgenographic
positioning
Roentgenography IV
Roentgenography IV lab
Elective

Emergency procedures
Emergency procedures lab
Adjusting procedures VI
Adjusting procedures VI
lab
Clinic I

*Quarter 9—Junior III*

Clinical diagnosis
Roentgenography V
Roentgenography V lab
Elective

Adjusting procedures VII
Adjusting procedures
VII lab
Philosophy IV
Clinic II

*Quarter 10—Senior I*

Neuromusculoskeletal
diagnosis
Neuromusculoskeletal
diagnosis lab
Case management

Clinical human behavior
Obstetrics and gynecology
Pediatrics
Febrile disorders
Clinic III

*Quarter 11—Senior II*

| | |
|---|---|
| Roentgenography V | Office procedures |
| Roentgenography V lab | Jurisprudence |
| Roentgenographic | Elective |
| pathology review | Clinic IV |
| Ethics | |

*Quarter 12—Senior III*

| | |
|---|---|
| Geriatrics | Philosophy V |
| Cardiovascular disorders | Clinical diagnosis seminar |
| Roentgenography VI | Elective |
| Roentgenography VI lab | Clinic V |

Table 7 shows a comparison of minimum class and clinic clock hours required by various colleges, as specified in their 1983 catalogs.

**TABLE 7. APPROXIMATE MODEL OF TOTAL COURSE
AND CLINIC HOURS**
(Subject to Change)

| | *Total class hours* | *Total clinic hours** | *Minimum Grand Total* |
|---|---|---|---|
| Cleveland (Kansas City) . . . | 3920 | 576 | 4496 |
| Cleveland (Los Angeles) . . . | 5640 | 560 | 5200 |
| Life—West . . . . . . . . . . . . | 4200 | 504 | 4704 |
| Logan . . . . . . . . . . . . . . . | 4365 | 1250 | 5615 |
| Los Angeles . . . . . . . . . . . | 3750 | 975 | 4725 |
| National . . . . . . . . . . . . . | 3750 | 1100 | 4850 |
| New York . . . . . . . . . . . . | 3936 | 1084 | 5020 |
| Northwestern . . . . . . . . . . | 4168 | 1222 | 5380 |
| Palmer . . . . . . . . . . . . . . | 3960 | 480 | 4440 |
| Parker . . . . . . . . . . . . . . | 3632 | 1008 | 4640 |
| Texas . . . . . . . . . . . . . . . | 4035 | 1044 | 5079 |
| Western States . . . . . . . . . | 3648 | 852 | 4500 |

*Frequently includes preceptorship.

## Typical Electives

Adjustive technics (elective)
Biofeedback
Biomechanics (advanced)
Dynamic reading
Hospital protocol
Hypnosis
Instrumentation (special)
Kinesiology
Meridian therapy
Nutritional therapeutics
Physiotherapy
Research planning and procedures
Sports-related disorders
Other special topics

## INSTRUCTIONAL ORGANIZATION

The curriculum for the Doctor of Chiropractic degree is typically divided into several divisions of instruction such as the Division of Basic Sciences, the Division of Clinical Sciences, the Division of Chiropractic, the Division of Research, and the Division of Postgraduate Education. Each division includes various departments that teach the required subject matter. In addition, a number of electives are offered to meet a student's particular interests. A general organizational structure is shown below:

## Division of Basic Sciences

*Department of Anatomy*

Angiology
Arthrology
Dissection
Embryology
Genesiology
Histology
Myology
Neurology
Osteology
Regional anatomy
Spinology
Splanchnology
Syndesmology
Topography

*Department of Physiology and Chemistry*

| | |
|---|---|
| Biochemistry | Physiology |
| Endrocrinology | Toxicology |
| Genetics | |

*Department of Pathology and Microbiology*

| | |
|---|---|
| Microbiology | Pathology |
| Micropathology | Public health and hygiene |

### Division of Clinical Sciences

*Department of Diagnosis and Clinical Practices*

| | |
|---|---|
| Allergic reactions | Hematology |
| Biophysics | Kinesiology |
| Cardiovascular disorders | Musculoskeletal disorders |
| Clinical laboratory diagnosis | Neurologic disorders |
| | Nutrition |
| Dermatology | Obstetrics |
| Dietetics | Orthopedic disorders |
| Electrocardiology | Pediatrics |
| Emergency health care | Physical diagnosis |
| Eye-ear-nose-throat disorders | Physical therapy |
| | Physical disorders |
| Febrile disorders | Respiratory disorders |
| Genitourinary disorders | Splanchnic disorders |
| Geriatrics | |
| Gynecologic disorders | |

*Department of Roentgenology*

| | |
|---|---|
| Patient positioning | Roentgenology |
| Roentgenographic diagnosis | X-ray physics |

## Division of Chiropractic

*Department of Principles and Technique*

| | |
|---|---|
| Adjusting procedures | Office management |
| Appendicular biomechanics | Palpation |
| | Patient relations |
| Appendicular orthopedics | Preceptorship program |
| Case management | Pharmacology |
| Chiropractic principles | Philosophy |
| Clinic management | Physiotherapy |
| Ethics | Psychiatry |
| First aid | Research methodology |
| Immunogenesis | Spinal biomechanics |
| Insurance relations | Spinal orthopedics |
| Jurisprudence | Terminology |
| Minor surgery | |

*Department of Clinical Practice*

## Division of Research

## Division of Postgraduate Education

## APPENDIX D

# TYPICAL TUITION AND FEES

Tuition, laboratory classes, and student activities fees are due and payable on registration day. Students must either pay the assessed fees in full before entering class or make prior arrangements with the college business office for payment of fees from loans and grants to be received during the semester.

Tuition and fees are subject to change at any time. As a general rule, costs will be adjusted once a year to be in effect for summer, fall, and spring terms of an entire academic year. New tuition and fee rates are usually announced in the spring prior to the beginning of the coming year.

Tuition and fees vary widely among the institutions. Some colleges incorporate many fees within the basic tuition fee, while others do not. Thus, careful analysis of each college's catalog is recommended. Table 8 shows the range of typical charges.

### Service Charges

There is a charge for any check submitted to the college that is not honored by the bank. In such cases, all subsequent payments to the college must in the form of a certified check or money order. In addition, the student will be required to pay a late payment fee. Students are also advised that they will be considered absent from class from the start of the trimester to the date of payment with the possibility of jeopardizing their continuance in the program if the hours lost are in excess of the allowance percentage.

### TABLE 8. RANGE OF TYPICAL TUITION AND FEES

| *Tuition and Fees* | *Range* |
| --- | --- |
| Tuition per trimester | $2200–2900 |
| or tuition per quarter | 1700–2200 |
| Tuition deposit (nonrefundable) | 25–350 |
| Fees: | |
| Application fee (usually nonrefundable) | 25–75 |
| Laboratory fees: | |
| Chemistry | 20–65 |
| Clinical | 30–65 |
| Dissection | 60–65 |
| First aid | 10–65 |
| Histology | 10–65 |
| Microbiology | 30–65 |
| Pathology | 15–65 |
| Physiology | 26–65 |
| Technic | 10–65 |
| Roentgenography | 30–65 |
| Intern clinic insurance (3rd & 4th academic year) | 25–30 |
| Student activities per trimester or quarter | 5–28 |
| Student health care fee per trimester or quarter | 13–cost |
| Library fee per trimester or quarter | 0–16 |
| Student/clinic identification and registration | 3–25 |
| Graduation and diploma fees | 25–150 |
| Transcripts: | |
| First transcript | 0–5 |
| Subsequent transcripts | 3–10 |
| Books/equipment per calendar year (variable) | 200–900 |
| Miscellaneous per trimester or quarter | 10–60 |

*Special Fees*

| | | |
|---|---:|---:|
| Late registration | $ | 10–100 |
| Late payment fee | | 10–50 |
| Returned check (NSF) | | 5–25 |
| Reinstatement fee | | 25–50 |
| Parking per trimester or quarter | | 0–10 |
| Make-up examinations, each | | 10–25 |
| Advanced standing compentency examination | | 15–20 |
| ID Replacement | | 5–10 |

## Payment Schedule

Tuition and fees must be paid in advance of the start of the trimester. Class admission cards will be provided at the time of registration. The student's name will not be admitted to the roster unless a class admission card has been issued. Special course tuition and fees are not refundable.

Registrations are validated when all fees have been paid and no outstanding indebtedness to the college exists. The privileges of the college are not available to the student until he or she has completed registration and the payment of all fees and tuition.

## Closing Remarks

The Boards of Trustees and the administration of each college reserve the right to make changes in policy, admission requirements, and tuition and fees, without notice or liability. Prospective students should contact those colleges in which they are interested for current and anticipated changes in policy.

# Chiropractic Oath

I do hereby affirm before God and these assembled witnesses that I will keep this oath and stipulation:

To hold in esteem and respect those who taught me this chiropractic healing art; to follow the methods of treatment which according to my ability and judgment I consider for the benefit of my patients; to abstain from whatever is deleterious and mischievous; to stand ready at all times to serve my fellow man without distinction of race, creed or color.

With purity I will pass my life and practice my art; I will at all times consider the patients under my care as of supreme importance; I will not spare myself in rendering them the help which I have been taught to give by my alma mater; I will keep inviolate all things revealed to me as a physician.

While I continue to keep this oath unviolated, may it be granted to me to enjoy life and the practice of the chiropractic healing art, respected by all men at all times.

Adopted by The Council on Chiropractic Education, January 1972

# VGM CAREER BOOKS

## OPPORTUNITIES IN

*Available in both
paperback and hardbound
editions*

Accounting Careers
Acting Careers
Advertising Careers
Airline Careers
Animal and Pet Care
Appraising Valuation Science
Architecture
Automotive Service
Banking
Beauty Culture
Biological Sciences
Book Publishing Careers
Broadcasting Careers
Building Construction Trades
Business Communication Careers
Business Management
Cable Television
Carpentry Careers
Chemical Engineering
Chemistry Careers
Child Care Careers
Chiropractic Health Care
Civil Engineering Careers
Commercial Art and Graphic
  Design
Computer Aided Design
  and Computer Aided Mfg.
Computer Science Careers
Counseling & Development
Dance
Data Processing Careers
Dental Care
Drafting Careers
Electrical Trades
Electronic and Electrical
  Engineering
Energy Careers
Engineering Technology Careers
Environmental Careers
Fashion Careers
Federal Government Careers
Film Careers
Financial Careers
Fire Protection Services
Fitness Careers
Food Services
Foreign Language Careers
Forestry Careers
Gerontology Careers
Government Service
Graphic Communications
Health and Medical Careers

High Tech Careers
Hospital Administration
Hotel & Motel Management
Industrial Design
Insurance Careers
Interior Design
Journalism Careers
Landscape Architecture
Law Careers
Law Enforcement and
  Criminal Justice
Library and Information
  Science
Machine Trades
Magazine Publishing Careers
Management
Marine & Maritime
Materials Science
Mechanical Engineering
Microelectronics
Modeling Careers
Music Careers
Nursing Careers
Nutrition Careers
Occupational Therapy
Office Occupations
Opticianry
Optometry
Packaging Science
Paralegal Careers
Paramedical Careers
Part-time & Summer Jobs
Personnel Management
Pharmacy Careers
Photography
Physical Therapy Careers
Podiatric Medicine
Printing Careers
Psychiatry
Psychology
Public Relations Careers
Real Estate
Recreation and Leisure
Refrigeration and
  Air Conditioning
Religious Service
Robotics Careers
Sales & Marketing
Secretarial Careers
Securities Industry
Sports & Athletics
Sports Medicine
State and Local Government
Teaching Careers
Technical Communications
Telecommunications

Theatrical Design
  & Production
Transportation
Travel Careers
Veterinary Medicine Careers
Vocational and Technical
  Careers
Word Processing
Writing Careers
Your Own Service Business

## WOMEN IN

Communications
Engineering
Finance
Government
Management
Science
Their Own Business

## CAREERS IN

Accounting
Business
Communications
Computers
Health Care
Science

## CAREER DIRECTORY

Occupational Outlook Handbook

## CAREER PLANNING

How to Get People to Do
  Things Your Way
How to Have a Winning
  Job Interview
How to Land a Better Job
How to Write a Winning
  Résumé
Life Plan
Planning Your Career Change
Planning Your Career of
  Tomorrow
Planning Your College
  Education
Planning Your Military Career
Planning Your Own Home
  Business
Planning Your Young Child's
  Education

## SURVIVAL GUIDES

High School Survival Guide
College Survival Guide

 **VGM Career Horizons**
A Division of National Textbook Company
4255 West Touhy Avenue
Lincolnwood, Illinois 60646-1975 U.S.A.

ANGLO-EUROPEAN COLLEGE OF CHIROPRACTIC